THE
EVERYTHING
PREGNANCY BOOK
4TH EDITION

Dear Reader,

When I was pregnant with my first child, I was overwhelmed by the sheer volume of pregnancy and childbirth information available, and completely underwhelmed by the available means to sort through it all. Everyone had advice for me, and it was usually some unsolicited nugget of wisdom passed along from a neighbor's third cousin. Although my health care providers were wonderful, they weren't present to answer those 2 A.M. "Was that a kick or heartburn?" questions, nor were they able to address more practical matters such as negotiating additional maternity leave or finding clothing that didn't look like it was from the Gymboree plus-size collection. In this spirit, I hope you find *The Everything® Pregnancy Book, 4th Edition*, a useful survival manual to get you through your next 9 months.

So, congratulations to you and your family for embarking on this grand adventure. As you adjust to the prospect of becoming a mom (or a repeat mom) and start to know that little person growing inside you, make sure you take time to savor your pregnancy. Nine months may seem like a long time, but as preparation for a lifetime of parenthood, it's merely a weekend seminar.

Sincerely,

Paula Ford-Martin

Welcome to the EVERYTHING® Series!

These handy, accessible books give you all you need to tackle a difficult project, gain a new hobby, comprehend a fascinating topic, prepare for an exam, or even brush up on something you learned back in school but have since forgotten.

You can choose to read an Everything® book from cover to cover or just pick out the information you want from our four useful boxes: e-ssentials, e-questions, e-facts, and e-alerts.

We give you everything you need to know on the subject, but throw in a lot of fun stuff along the way, too.

We now have more than 400 Everything® books in print, spanning such wide-ranging categories as weddings, pregnancy, cooking, music instruction, foreign language, crafts, pets, New Age, and so much more. When you're done reading them all, you can finally say you know Everything®!

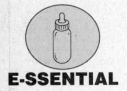

E-SSENTIAL

Answers to
common questions

E-QUESTION

Important snippets
of information

E-FACT

Urgent
warnings

E-ALERT!

Quick
handy tips

PUBLISHER Karen Cooper

DIRECTOR OF ACQUISITIONS AND INNOVATION Paula Munier

MANAGING EDITOR, EVERYTHING® SERIES Lisa Laing

COPY CHIEF Casey Ebert

ASSISTANT PRODUCTION EDITOR Melanie Cordova

ACQUISITIONS EDITOR Brett Palana-Shanahan

SENIOR DEVELOPMENT EDITOR Brett Palana-Shanahan

EDITORIAL ASSISTANT Ross Weisman

EVERYTHING® SERIES COVER DESIGNER Erin Alexander

LAYOUT DESIGNERS Erin Dawson, Michelle Roy Kelly, Elisabeth Lariviere, Denise Wallace

Visit the entire Everything® series at *www.everything.com*

THE
EVERYTHING®
Pregnancy
Book

4TH EDITION

All you need to get you through the most
important nine months of your life!

PAULA FORD-MARTIN
TECHNICAL REVIEW BY VINCENT IANNELLI, MD

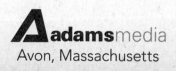
Avon, Massachusetts

For the best kids a mom could ask for—
Cassie, Kate, Chris, and John

An Everything® Series Book.
Everything® and everything.com® are registered trademarks of F+W Media, Inc.

Published by Adams Media, a division of F+W Media, Inc.
57 Littlefield Street, Avon, MA 02322 U.S.A.
www.adamsmedia.com

ISBN 10: 1-4405-2851-9
ISBN 13: 978-1-4405-2851-4
eISBN 10: 1-4405-3035-1
eISBN 13: 978-1-4405-3035-7

Printed in the United States of America.

10 9 8 7 6 5 4 3 2

Library of Congress Cataloging-in-Publication Data
is available from the publisher.

This book is available at quantity discounts for bulk purchases.
For information, please call 1-800-289-0963.

Contents

Acknowledgments

My heartfelt gratitude and love go out to my husband, Tim, for his support, encouragement, and help throughout this project (the "firstborn" of our marriage). And as always, I owe a big thank you to agent Barb Doyen and to editor Brett Shanahan for their guidance and expertise during the gestation and delivery of the fourth edition of this book.

Top 10 Things Every Pregnant Woman Should Know

1. Morning sickness doesn't just happen in the morning.

2. Trust your instincts—what worked for your neighbor, friend, or sister isn't necessarily what's right for you.

3. A birth plan can help you and your partner work toward the labor and delivery experience you want.

4. Things don't always go according to plan, but being prepared for the possibilities can make the detours easier to handle.

5. Taking 600 micrograms of folic acid during pregnancy can dramatically reduce your risk of having a baby with neural tube defects.

6. A due date is a suggestion, not a contractual obligation.

7. Career and family are not mutually exclusive.

8. Federal legislation provides specific protections against pregnancy discrimination in the workplace.

9. Alcohol and tobacco in pregnancy can have serious health repercussions for your baby.

10. Stress can be hard on the health of you and your baby; make sure you have a support system for both pregnancy and new motherhood.

Introduction

YOUR MOTHER ALWAYS SAID, "You'll understand when you have kids of your own." And as much as you may hate to admit it, she's right. Being a mom starts the day you find out you're no longer a solo act; suddenly responsibility means more than remembering when the cat needs shots and getting the oil changed every 3,000 miles. Pregnancy initiates you into an empathic sisterhood of women who can be a source of inspiration, support, and advice throughout pregnancy and beyond.

It's a big club—more than 4.1 million American women gave birth in 2009 alone—but it's surprisingly intimate in the knowledge of the trials and tribulations of motherhood. Never again will you roll your eyes at a toddler throwing a tantrum in the grocery store or tap your fingers impatiently at that woman taking forever to load her kids in the car and pull out of your parking space. Mothers understand that pregnancy and parenting require patience, love, and compassion.

Pregnancy also means preparing for a whole new lifestyle. You and your significant other will no longer pass as "couples only"; your free time will focus on parks and playgroups rather than on dinner and a show. If you already have children, the challenges and joys of new sibling relationships lie ahead. And your husband or partner will be exploring his new role as a dad and learning the ropes of child care. It's an exciting time, but as with any unfamiliar venture, pregnancy and the prospect of this completely dependent tiny person can inspire anxiety and, yes, even fear. Are you eating the right foods? Is your morning run bad for your baby? Will your child develop your grandfather's diabetes? In true motherly style, you've started worrying about your baby's well-being already.

Of course, your health care provider is the best source of information for specific medical questions about your pregnancy. But even the most dedicated doctor can't be at your disposal 24/7. This book is designed as your personal pregnancy assistant—an essential educational reference for your pregnancy concerns and a guide for more practical matters like career considerations, car seats, and family budgets. It's also an invaluable resource for helping you plan a birth experience you'll treasure.

Most important, this book encourages an open dialogue with your health care provider. Your doctor or midwife can provide medical care and expert advice, but ultimately you must manage your health care for yourself. That means reading up, asking questions, and making sure you're satisfied with the answers. After all, you wouldn't let your financial planner do whatever he pleases with your money without your providing some input and approval. Yet many women don't feel they have a right to bother their doctors with their questions about a much more precious investment—their child.

You'll make many critical decisions throughout your pregnancy, from pursuing diagnostic testing and genetic counseling to choosing your labor and delivery preferences. Educating yourself allows you to make informed choices and to make the most of your time with your doctor or midwife. Most health care providers are more than willing to answer your questions; patients who do their homework demonstrate their commitment to healthy pregnancies and make their providers' jobs easier in the long run. But remember, communication is key. Your questions will go unanswered if you fail to ask them.

Enjoy this special time, and consider this book a key part of your support team. The highly coveted mother's intuition is usually made, not born, and will develop in time as you become better acquainted with your growing baby and learn more about this exciting journey called *pregnancy and parenthood*.

Getting Ready

Pregnancy is a time of big changes for your family, for your body, and for your emotional equilibrium. There's a lot to learn as you prepare for parenthood—both physically and mentally—so be patient with yourself. Finding balance, keeping yourself healthy, and choosing a health care provider who will support you in this endeavor are crucial to creating the best possible environment for baby, both in and outside the womb.

So You're Pregnant . . .

You just found out you're pregnant. Perhaps you've been trying for just a few months, or maybe for a few years. There's also a good chance this baby has taken you by surprise; about half of all pregnancies among American women are unintended. Planned or unplanned, pregnancy stirs up a wide spectrum of emotions. You may be on cloud nine and picking out nursery patterns, or you may be in a state of shock wondering how you're going to handle it all.

Relax. You're normal. Everyone reacts differently to the joys and jeopardies of pregnancy. Preparing yourself for the road ahead is the best way to overcome your fears and get a realistic picture of what pregnancy, and motherhood, entails. So ask questions, read up, take classes, and talk to friends and family who have been there. There's no such thing as too much information when it comes to your (and your baby's) health.

A Different Kind of Family Tree

Even if you and your partner are in perfect health, you may have a family history of chronic illness or medical disorders that could impact the health of your unborn child. Your health care provider will ask you questions about your ethnic and racial heritage and family background (and that of the baby's father) to screen for medical conditions for which your child may be at risk. Having the most-complete and most-accurate information possible will help her determine what screening tests, if any, you ought to consider.

In addition to the medical history of your partner and yourself, as well as that of any children you already have, you should gather all known health information going back two generations (that is, information on your and your partner's parents and siblings, along with that of your second-degree relatives, including grandparents and blood-related aunts and uncles). Any additional information you have about medical conditions further back in your family tree should also be brought to your provider's attention.

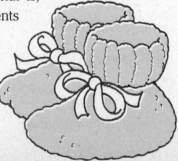

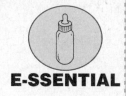

Don't rely too much on the health histories in family adoption records. There is no guarantee that the healthy twenty-year-old who gave birth didn't develop major medical problems later in life. In many cases the original adoption information includes no medical history beyond a brief physical indicator at the time of the adoption (for example, mother "appeared to be in good health").

Parents-to-be who were adopted may have little to no information on their birth families. If you'd like to pursue access to your health history, your first step is to know the law. Some states allow nonidentifying (non-ID) information to be given out. Non-ID is information about the adoption excluding any information that would enable you to identify the people involved. In many cases the non-ID information will include some medical and social history of the birth parents, although in some states this information is only voluntary and may not be available.

If you have a history of health problems or miscarriage and your doctor feels more family background would be valuable, many states provide a system by which an adoptee can petition the court to get adoption records opened or unsealed.

Keep in mind that only 3 percent of American infants are born with a birth defect, only a portion of which are thought to have a genetic component. In many cases of inherited diseases, a complex interaction of both genetic and environmental factors is required to trigger the condition. If your provider determines you are at risk for passing along a medical problem to your child, she may refer you to a genetic counselor for analysis of your risk factors and a discussion of options for additional testing or another appropriate course of action.

Finding a Health Care Provider

Even if you have a model pregnancy, you will be seeing a lot of your health care provider over the next 9 months. The American College of Obstetricians and Gynecologists (ACOG) recommends that women see their providers every 4 weeks through the first 28 weeks of pregnancy (about the first 7 months). After week 28, the visits will increase to once every 2 to 3 weeks until week 36, after which you'll be paying your doctor or midwife a weekly visit until your baby arrives. If you have any conditions that put you in a high-risk category (for example, diabetes, history of preterm labor), your provider may want to see you more frequently to monitor your progress.

The Options

So, who should guide you on this odyssey? If you currently see a gynecologist or family practice doctor who also has an obstetric practice, he or she may be a good choice. If you don't have that choice or would like to explore your options, consider:

- **An ob-gyn:** An obstetrician and gynecologist (ob-gyn) is a medical doctor (MD) who has received specialized training in women's health and reproductive medicine.
- **A perinatologist:** If you have a chronic health condition, you may see a perinatologist—an ob-gyn who specializes in overseeing high-risk pregnancies.
- **A midwife:** Certified nurse-midwives are licensed to practice in all fifty states. They provide patient-focused care throughout pregnancy, labor, and delivery.
- **A nurse practitioner:** A nurse practitioner (NP) is a registered nurse (RN) with advanced medical education and training (at minimum, a master's degree).
- **Combined practice:** Some obstetric practices blend midwives, NPs, and MDs, with the choice (sometimes the requirement) of seeing one or more of these throughout your pregnancy.

Networking and Referrals

Finding Dr. Right may seem like a monumental task; after all, this is the person to whom you're entrusting your pregnancy and your childbirth.

Unless you're paying completely out-of-pocket for all prenatal care, labor, and delivery expenses, your first consideration is probably your health insurance coverage. If you are part of a managed-care organization, your insurer may require that you see someone within its provider network. Getting a current copy of the network directory, if one is available, can help you narrow down your choices by coverage and location.

E-QUESTION

What is a doula, and is it too early to get one?
A doula is a pregnancy-and-birth support person whose job is to provide emotional assistance to both the mom-to-be and her family. Doulas can assist you at any point in pregnancy, from preconception to postpartum issues.

Many women choose a physician solely for logistical reasons (for example, insurance coverage or office location). Although money and convenience are important factors, these won't mean much if you aren't happy with the care you receive and with the role your health care provider will ultimately play in your pregnancy and birth. Whether this is your first or your fifth, this pregnancy is a one-time-only event. You deserve the best support in seeing it through. Talk to the experts—girlfriends and other women you know and trust—and get referrals. Be aware that not everyone looks for the same thing in a health care provider; what one woman can't stand may not be a big deal to you. With this in mind, you might find it more efficient to limit your survey to friends and family you know well rather than asking every mother you encounter.

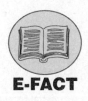

E-FACT

Need a referral? The American College of Obstetricians and Gynecologists can help you find a physician in your area (all ACOG fellows are board-certified ob-gyns). Search their membership at *www.acog.org* (click on "Find an Ob/Gyn"). To find a nurse-midwife, contact the American College of Nurse-Midwives at *www.midwife.org* (click on "Find a Midwife").

If you've just moved to a new area or simply don't know any moms or moms-to-be, there are other referral options available. The licensing authority in your area (the state or county medical board) can typically provide you with references for local practitioners. You may also try the patient services department or labor and delivery programs of nearby hospitals and/or birthing centers.

Ask the Right Questions

Once you've collected names and phone numbers, narrowed down your list of potential providers, and verified that they accept (and are accepted by) your health insurance plan, it's time to do some legwork. Sit down with your partner and talk about your biggest questions, concerns, and expectations. Then compile a list of provider "interview questions." Some issues to consider:

✓ **What are the costs and payment options?** If your health plan doesn't provide full coverage, find out how much the remaining fees will run and whether installment plans are available.

✓ **Who will deliver my baby?** Will the doctor or midwife you select deliver your child, or might it be another provider in the practice, depending on when the baby arrives? If your provider works alone, find out who covers his patients during vacations and emergencies.

✓ **Whom will I see during office visits?** Since group practices typically share delivery responsibilities, you might want to ask about rotating your prenatal appointments among all the providers in the group so that you'll see a familiar face in the delivery room when the big day arrives.

✓ **What is the provider's philosophy on routine IVs, episiotomies, labor induction, pain relief, and other interventions in the birth process?** If you have certain expectations regarding medical interventions during labor and delivery, you should lay them out now.

✓ **What hospital or birthing center will I go to?** Find out where the provider has hospital privileges, and obtain more information on that facility's programs and policies. Is a neonatal unit available if problems arise after the baby's birth? Many hospitals offer expectant parents the opportunity to tour their labor and delivery rooms.

✓ **What is the provider's policy on birth plans?** Will the provider work with you to create and, more important, to follow a birth plan? Will the plan be signed and become part of your permanent chart in case he or she is off duty during the birth?

✓ **How are phone calls handled if I have a health concern or question?** Most obstetric practices have some sort of triage (prioritizing) system in place for patients' phone calls. Ask how quickly calls are returned and what system the practice has in place for handling night and weekend patient calls.

Some providers have the staff to answer these sorts of inquiries over the phone, while others might schedule a face-to-face appointment with your prospective doctor or midwife. Either way, make sure that all your questions are answered to your satisfaction so that you can make a fully informed choice.

Comfort and Communication

As with any good relationship, communication is essential between patients and their providers. Does the provider encourage your questions, answer them thoroughly, and really listen to your concerns? Does he make sure all your questions are answered before concluding the appointment? Are the nursing and administrative staff attentive to patients' needs and willing to answer questions as well?

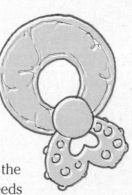

Good health care is a partnership or, more accurately, a team effort. Although ultimately you call the shots (it's your body and your baby, after all), your provider serves as your coach and trainer, giving you the support and training you need to reach the finish line. If your doctor doesn't listen to your needs, she likely won't be able to meet them. But also remember that communication works both ways. Your provider has likely been around the block a few times and has a wealth of useful information to offer you, particularly if you're a rookie at this baby game.

E-ALERT!

When you phone potential providers, pay close attention to how the support staff handle your calls. If the receptionist is rushed or rude or you're put on perpetual hold, that could signal a problem. Midwife and obstetric practices are notoriously busy, but a competent office staff will be both polite and reasonably timely with patient inquiries.

Although experience, education, and practice philosophy are key considerations in selecting a health care provider, your comfort is equally important. Is the doctor warm and compassionate, cold and humorless, outgoing and chatty, or reserved and distant? Even with a short introductory phone call or appointment, you should be able to get a feel for your potential provider's bedside manner. Is it a personality style you can effectively deal with for the next 9 months? If you're regaled with bad jokes or mind-numbingly boring clinical explanations at the doctor's office, just imagine how you'll feel hearing it in the delivery room.

Gender may also be an issue for you. Some women feel more at ease with a female physician. Making an issue of gender may seem silly or, at worst, discriminatory and hypocritical. The subject is serious enough to merit a number of clinical studies and patient surveys in medical literature, with results both for and against forming a clear gender preference. Some reasons given for choosing a woman doctor include communication style and the fact that the physician may have been through pregnancy herself.

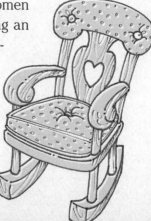

Other women may find that they prefer a male doctor for various reasons. The bottom line is that you are the one who has to live with your provider choice for the next 9 months, and to spend it feeling awkward, stressed, and inhibited—emotions that can ultimately have a negative effect on your pregnancy—is not healthy. Whatever your choice, make sure it's one you'll be comfortable with.

Smoking Cessation

You don't need anyone to tell you that cigarettes are bad for you. If you are a smoker, you've probably tried to stop, possibly more than once. It's not an easy endeavor, but now you have special motivation to quit and make it stick. In addition to the health risks smoking exposes you to, such as cardiovascular disease, lung cancer, and high blood pressure, it can also have dire consequences for your baby.

According to the U.S. Surgeon General, women who smoke are at increased risk for ectopic pregnancies and stillbirth, as well as premature birth, premature rupture of membranes (PROM), placenta previa, placental abruption, and intrauterine growth restriction (IUGR). The dangers continue after birth, with an increased risk of sudden infant death syndrome (SIDS), low birth weight, heart and other birth defects, asthma, colic, and childhood obesity. Even environmental exposure to tobacco smoke in pregnancy can be detrimental; secondhand smoke causes a slightly increased risk of IUGR, low birth weight, and SIDS. Cigarettes take a toll on the pocketbook as well; neonatal care–costs attributable to smoking account for more than $360 million annually.

E-ALERT!

The antidepressant bupropion is prescribed for smoking cessation. There is a lack of well-controlled human studies that ensure safe use in pregnancy, but potential benefits of the drug for some pregnant women may outweigh the risks. Your doctor should oversee the use of any drug or nicotine replacement therapy (NRT) product to ensure safe use.

If you're a smoker, ideally you will kick the habit in the planning stages of your pregnancy. However, the good news is that even if you're pregnant and still smoking, quitting now can make a big difference to your baby's health. Women who stop smoking in the first trimester of pregnancy greatly reduce the risk of IUGR for their children. For women who have difficulty quitting, nicotine replacement therapies—such as gum, patches, or inhalers—may be an option. Although these products are now available without a prescription, be sure to ask your doctor if you are considering their use. You should know that the safety and effectiveness of NRT in pregnancy has not been extensively tested, and animal studies have indicated that nicotine exposure in the womb may cause later breathing problems in offspring. However, for the mother-to-be who smokes heavily and is not able to stop through traditional cessation programs, the use of these products is preferable to cigarettes because they do not contain carbon monoxide or any of the other hundreds of toxic chemicals contained in cigarette smoke.

Exercising Your Body

Women who work out regularly or participate in sports are often worried about whether they can continue their routine with a baby on board. In most cases, exercise is not only allowed; it's encouraged. ACOG recommends 30 minutes of moderate exercise activity daily for women who are pregnant (excluding high-risk pregnancies). All pregnant women, especially those in high-risk pregnancies and those who were inactive prior to pregnancy, should speak with their physician about exercise options.

Vigorous team sports that pose a risk of injury should be avoided (for example, basketball or soccer). Scuba diving is not advised because of the risk of decompression sickness. However, swimming, walking, and cycling are ideal ways to stay fit. Your local YMCA or community health center may also offer exercise programs geared toward the prenatal set.

Always stay well-hydrated when you work out, and try to confine exercise to the coolest parts of the day in the summer months. An excessive rise in core body temperature (hyperthermia), particularly in the first trimester, has been associated with birth defects. If you feel yourself getting warmer than is comfortable, stop your exercise routine and cool down.

Using Medications

Medication use in pregnancy is a thorny issue. There is simply not enough long-term clinical data available on most drugs to provide a 100 percent guarantee of their safety. Ideally, you should avoid all prescription and over-the-counter drugs, except for your prenatal supplements, throughout pregnancy. However, that's an unrealistic expectation given that two-thirds of all pregnant women take one or more prescription drugs at some point in their pregnancy. And if you have a chronic disease, such as diabetes, schizophrenia, or HIV, you have little choice but to continue your treatment.

Since 1979, the U.S. Food and Drug Administration (FDA) has used a classification system for drugs based on the degree of known risk that a medication presents to a fetus—known as *categories A, B, C, and X.* As of mid-2011, the agency was finalizing a new rule that would eliminate these categories and replace them with detailed drug labeling that outlines the safety of drugs to mother and developing child in pregnancy and lactation. You can also visit the U.S. National Library of Medicine's Drugs and Lactation Database at *www.nlm.nih.gov/pubs/factsheets/lactmedfs.html* for more information.

When deciding whether or not to take a drug in pregnancy, the consequences of not taking a medication should be considered. Do the benefits of the drug outweigh the risks to the mother and/or fetus? Can a safer medication be substituted temporarily? Or can the drug be temporarily stopped during the period of time it is known to potentially harm the fetus? With close observation, well-researched prescribing, and careful dosing, the use of many medications can proceed safely when necessary.

Sometimes women decide to self-treat colds and other illnesses with dietary supplements and herbal and botanical remedies in pregnancy, mistakenly assuming that medicine from a botanical source is inherently safe for their fetus. Remember: natural doesn't necessarily mean harmless; herbs can be potent medicinal substances. Always check with your care provider before taking anything medicinal—herbal or otherwise.

On Your Mind

Although physical wellness and mental health are often perceived as two separate things, the truth is that the mind and body are inextricably linked and what impacts one usually affects the other as well. This connection is particularly strong in pregnancy as the rapid physical changes taking place alter the biochemical balance of the body and brain. Pregnancy is also a precursor to one of the biggest life-changing events there is—the arrival of a baby—and that alone is enough to stir up new and unexpected feelings.

Emotional Health

The hormonal changes that occur in pregnancy can have you feeling weepy one minute and irritable the next. And the emotions you experience, especially the negative ones, can be detrimental to your growing child. Depression, stress, and anxiety may alter your eating and sleeping patterns, robbing you and baby of the nutrients and rest you need. Clinical studies have found that depression and stress also have a direct impact on fetal growth and infant development.

E-FACT

If you're feeling hopeless, sad, or tired; having trouble sleeping; or losing interest in things that once gave you pleasure, you may be experiencing antepartum depression. Research has linked depression during pregnancy to preterm delivery, lower birth weight, developmental problems in infancy, and a 50 percent chance of developing postpartum depression. Don't wait; talk to your provider about treatment options today.

If you are feeling blue, you aren't alone; one in ten women experiences depressive symptoms at some point in her pregnancy. Yet women frequently feel guilty that they are feeling so bad during a period of their lives that is supposed to be joyful, and for that reason many do not seek professional help.

Keeping Stress in Check

Pregnancy is a stressful time. A lot of it is positive, exciting stress as you plan for the baby. But you may also be feeling the pressures of impending financial and family responsibilities, fears of labor and delivery, and new career challenges. Trying to keep up with a hectic prepregnancy schedule as your body grows to a very large and unwieldy size is also a sure-fire way to stress out. In high enough amounts, the stress hormone *cortisol* can cross the placental barrier and impact neuromuscular and brain development in the fetus. That's why it's essential to take time out for yourself to decompress throughout your pregnancy.

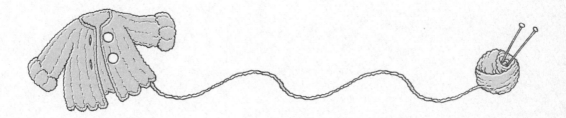

Month 1

During the first trimester of pregnancy, which lasts approximately 14 weeks from the first day of your last menstrual period, your body is hard at work forming one of the most intricate and complex works of nature. By the end of your first official month of pregnancy (6 weeks after your last menstrual period, but 4 weeks since conception), your developing child will have grown an astonishing 10,000 times in size since fertilization.

Baby This Month

Making its longest journey until the big move 9 months from now, your developing baby (at this point called a *zygote*, or *fertilized ovum*) travels from the Fallopian tube into the uterus (womb). After fertilization, the zygote begins a process of rapid cell division, and by day 4 it has formed a small, solid cluster of cells known as a *morula* (after *moris*, Latin for *mulberry*). The morula finishes the trip down the Fallopian tube, reaching the uterus about 3 or 4 days after fertilization.

The Blastocyst

By the fifth or sixth day, your baby takes on its third name change in less than a week as the morula grows to a blastocyst. The blastocyst contains two distinct cell layers with a cavity at the center. The inner layer will evolve into the embryo, and the outer layer will develop into the placental membranes—the amnion and the chorion. Within days, the blastocyst nestles into the nutrient-rich lining of your uterus (the endometrium) as implantation begins, about 1 week after conception. Wispy fingers of tissue called *chorionic villi* from the chorion layer will anchor the blastocyst firmly to your uterine wall, where they will begin to build a network of blood vessels. These villi are the start of the placenta, a spongy, oval-shaped structure that will feed the fetus (via the umbilical cord) with maternal nutrients and oxygen throughout pregnancy.

The Embryo

About 15 days after conception, the blastocyst officially becomes an embryo. Next to the embryo floats the yolk sac, a cluster of blood vessels that provide blood for the embryo at this early stage until the placenta takes over. The embryo is surrounded by a watertight sac called the *amnion* (*amniotic sac*). The amniotic fluid that fills the sac provides a warm and weightless environment for your developing baby. It also serves as a sort of embryo airbag (in this case, fluid bag), protecting baby from the bumps and bustle of your daily routine. Nature efficiently double-bags your baby, surrounding the embryo and the amnion with a second membrane called the *chorion*.

During these first 4 weeks of development, your embryo has laid the groundwork for most of its major organ systems. As month 1 draws to a close, baby's heart is beating (although you won't be able to hear it for several weeks yet), lung buds have appeared, and construction of the gastrointestinal system and liver is well under way. The neural tube, the basis of the baby's central nervous system, has developed, and the forebrain, midbrain, and hindbrain are defined. The embryo is starting to look more like a person, too. The first layer of skin has appeared, facial features are surfacing, and arm and leg buds—complete with the beginnings of feet and hands—are visible. It's an amazing list of accomplishments considering your baby is about the size of a raisin (less than ¼ inch long).

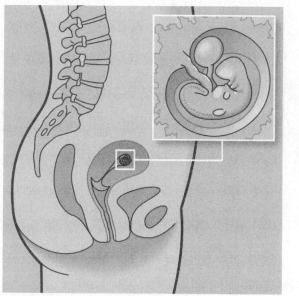

Now an embryo, your baby at 1 month gestation

Your Body This Month

From your tired and anxious mind to your busy bladder, all of your body's systems may seem to be in overdrive during these early days of pregnancy. The first thing you will notice is the absence of your monthly menstrual period—in many cases, this is what tipped you off to your pregnancy in the first place. Your embryo is secreting the human chorionic gonadotropin (hCG) hormone into your system. In addition to interrupting menstruation, hCG signals the ovaries to produce the hormone progesterone until week 8 of pregnancy, when the placenta takes over production.

Your Body Changes

At this point in your pregnancy, you might not notice any significant changes in shape and size. Although you aren't menstruating, you feel slightly bloated, and your waistband may begin to feel a bit snug. Your breasts may also start to increase in size, and the areolae around your nipples may enlarge and darken. No period? Bigger breasts? This baby is doing wonders for you already! Now for the cloud around that silver lining: fuller breasts are often more tender in pregnancy (although a supportive sports bra can help).

E-FACT

Some women experience minor vaginal blood flow, called *spotting*, as the embryo implants itself into the uterine wall. Because of the timing—1 week to 10 days after ovulation—it's often mistaken for the beginning of the menstrual period. The spotting, which usually lasts only a day or two, is pink to brown and may be accompanied by minor cramps.

You may also experience another hormonal side effect: increased vaginal secretions similar to those you get premenstrually. These typically last throughout pregnancy and may actually worsen in the third trimester. Normal vaginal secretions in pregnancy are clear to white in color, mucus-like, and both odor- and pain-free. If you experience discharge that is thick, foulsmelling, off-color, or accompanied by itching, blood, or pain, contact your health care provider immediately to rule out infection or other problems.

What You Feel Like

Building a baby is hard work, and even though it's early in the process, it isn't unusual to feel tired and rundown right now. If at all possible, try to grab a nap during the day. If that isn't feasible because of a full-time job or young children at home, make early bedtime a priority. Although it may run contrary to your nature to be sleeping away the daylight hours when you could be accomplishing one of the seventy-five things on your to-do list, thinking of it as a naptime for baby might help. Once you start down the long road of sleepless nights that new motherhood brings, you'll be longing for the days of early bedtimes and frequent naps!

You may also find yourself spending more and more time in the bathroom. You are urinating more frequently due to high levels of progesterone, which relaxes your bladder muscles. Unfortunately, frequent urination is one symptom that will likely remain with you throughout pregnancy as your baby grows and the uterus exerts more and more pressure on your bladder. And although constipation typically doesn't become a common pregnancy complaint for several months yet, if you're taking iron supplements you may be experiencing problems now.

Your cardiovascular system is undergoing big changes right now as it adjusts to meet baby's growing demand for the oxygen and nutrients your blood is carrying. Circulating pregnancy hormones dilate (expand) your blood vessels to accommodate an eventual 50-percent increase in blood volume. Your cardiac output, a measure of how hard your heart is working to pump blood, increases by 30 to 50 percent, whereas your blood pressure drops. This is why you may find yourself feeling faint. If you feel dizzy or lightheaded, sit down, or lie down on your side, as soon as possible. Try not to lie flat on your back, particularly later in pregnancy, because the pressure your uterus places on both the aorta and the inferior vena cava (two of the large blood vessels that help keep oxygen circulating to you and baby) will actually make the dizziness worse.

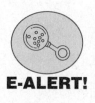

E-ALERT!

If episodes of fainting or dizziness persist or are accompanied by abdominal pain or bleeding, contact your health care provider immediately. They could be symptoms of ectopic (tubal) pregnancy, a potentially fatal condition in which implantation occurs outside the endometrial lining of the uterus (for example, in the Fallopian tubes).

And then there's the most notorious of all pregnancy symptoms—morning sickness. Referred to by clinicians as *nausea and vomiting of pregnancy* (NVP), up to 80 percent of women experience one or both of these symptoms at some point in their pregnancy. As you may know all too well by now, the more accurate term is morning, noon, and night sickness; NVP can happen at any time and strikes with varying intensity. Many women find that their stomach starts to settle as the first trimester draws to a close (anywhere from week 12 to week 16), but for others the queasiness persists throughout the entire pregnancy.

At Your Doctor Visit

Set up your first prenatal care visit as soon as you know you are pregnant. For now through the 7th month, you'll be seeing your provider on a monthly basis (unless you are considered high-risk, in which case you may have more frequent appointments). If you're seeing a new doctor or midwife, expect your initial visit to be a bit longer than subsequent checkups because you'll be asked to fill out medical history forms and insurance paperwork. Some providers will send you these materials in advance so that you can complete them at home.

Your provider will ask plenty of questions about your health history and the pregnancy symptoms you have been experiencing. Make sure that you take advantage of this initial appointment to ask about issues that are on your mind as well. In addition, you will undergo a thorough physical examination, give a urine sample (the first of many), and have blood drawn for routine lab work. If you haven't had a Pap smear within the last year, your provider may also take a vaginal swab of cells scraped from your cervix for this purpose.

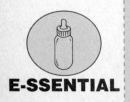

E-SSENTIAL

Remember, the dad-to-be is in this pregnancy, too. By all means, bring him to the doctor with you. In addition to providing moral support, he probably has just as many questions about the baby as you do. He can also help you remember the things your provider tells you that seem to promptly exit your brain as soon as you leave the examining room.

Your provider will probably supply you with educational brochures and pamphlets on prenatal care, nutrition, office policies, and other important issues. There will be a lot of new information to absorb, so don't feel as though you have to study everything on the spot. However, do take everything home to read and refer to later.

Confirming Your Pregnancy

Today's home pregnancy tests are highly sensitive (many claim a 99 percent or higher accuracy rate) and provide many women with a convenient and private way to confirm their pregnancy. However, juggling sticks, strips, and tiny plastic cups while trying to decode the magic-answer window does leave some room for operator error.

If your provider hasn't yet officially confirmed your pregnancy with a lab test, he will do so at this first visit, typically with a urine test, although a blood (serum) test may be used. The pregnancy test measures the amount of hCG in your system. Blood tests may be performed in cases where a urine test is negative but pregnancy is still suspected (usually in the early weeks of pregnancy) or when an abnormal pregnancy may be suspected.

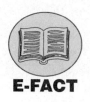

E-FACT

Because your urine will not start to contain hCG until after the embryo is implanted in the endometrial lining of the uterine wall, a home test will not always detect your pregnancy as early as claimed. An estimated 10 percent of clinical pregnancies are undetectable when using a urine hCG test on the first day of a missed menstrual period.

Estimating Your Due Date

Although pregnancy lasts approximately 280 days or about 9 calendar months, your estimated date of delivery (EDD) is based on a 10-lunar-month pregnancy. Each lunar month is four 7-day weeks. Why lunar months instead of following a good old-fashioned calendar? Lunar months are based on a 28-day menstrual cycle, which is considered the average cycle length.

It's important to remember that most providers determine gestational age (how far along you are) from the first day of your last menstrual period (LMP). This means that you are officially 2 weeks pregnant at the moment of conception. How's that for an existential twist? Of course, if your cycle is longer or shorter than 28 days, or if you have an irregular menstrual period, or if you're hazy on the date of your LMP, the EDD could be harder to pinpoint.

To avoid confusion, your provider probably makes good use of the printed EDD charts in her office. However, if you do have a regular 28-day cycle, you can figure out your own EDD by taking the date of your last period, counting 3 months back, and then adding 7 days. For example, if your last period began on September 1, you would go back through August, July, and June, to June 1. Then add 7 days to come up with an estimated due date of June 8 (of the following year). An alternate method is to count 280 days (40 weeks) from the first day of your last period.

Prenatal Vitamins

Although some experts question whether you need to supplement a well-balanced diet with a vitamin and mineral dosage, most practitioners feel that a daily prenatal supplement can't hurt and in many cases will benefit you and your developing fetus. A basic prenatal supplement contains vitamins A, D, E, C, B_1, B_2, B_6, B_{12}, calcium, copper, iron, magnesium, zinc, and folic acid (other vitamins and minerals may be included). It is recommended that you take a minimum daily dose of 600 micrograms (mcg) of folic acid, plus other essential nutrients such as iron and calcium, to prevent neural tube defects in the first trimester. Some women find prenatal supplements, which are the rough equivalent of a horse pill, tough to swallow (literally). And if you're experiencing morning sickness, you may find them hard to keep down. Try experimenting with different brands and formulations; there are chewable and flavored versions now on the market. Your provider probably has a roomful of samples for the asking, so request some freebies if they aren't offered.

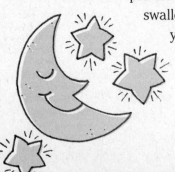

Learning the Ropes

At each appointment you'll provide a urine sample, have a weigh-in, and get your blood pressure taken. Other diagnostic and screening tests may be administered throughout pregnancy. Once you're in the examining room, you may or may not have to disrobe, depending on your provider's policy and how far along you are. For your first prenatal visit, you will probably don a gown for a full physical exam. Later, some providers will simply have you move your clothing aside for a quick belly check and measure, while others prefer a more thorough examination (for example, checking your heart rate, examining your feet for swelling).

When to Call the Doctor, Day or Night

At your first appointment, your provider may discuss how patients' phone calls are handled both during the day and after hours. Frequently, obstetric practices use a triage system in which the receptionist or intake coordinator answers and prioritizes calls and has a nurse, midwife, or physician return them in order of urgency. If your doctor is in the office and you feel more comfortable speaking with her directly (and don't mind waiting a little longer for your answer, if necessary), be sure to make your preference known when you call.

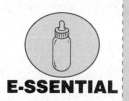

E-SSENTIAL

Get to know the support staff in your provider's office. Not only will it make your visits a more pleasant experience; it also provides you with an invaluable personal contact when you're trying to squeeze in an unexpected appointment, experiencing insurance difficulties, or having trouble reaching your doctor.

Usually an answering service will pick up after-hours calls and will page the doctor or midwife on duty, who will then return your call. In most group practices, providers take turns covering nights and weekends, so you will get a call back from the on-call practitioner. If you aren't given any guidelines for reaching staff after hours, make sure you ask.

Call your doctor immediately if you experience any of the following symptoms:

- ✓ Abdominal pain and/or cramping
- ✓ Fluid or blood leaking from the vagina
- ✓ Abnormal vaginal discharge (for example, foul-smelling, green, or yellow)
- ✓ Painful urination
- ✓ Severe headache
- ✓ Impaired vision (for example, spots, blurring)
- ✓ Fever over 101°F
- ✓ Chills
- ✓ Excessive swelling of face and/or body
- ✓ Severe and unrelenting vomiting and/or diarrhea

Some women hesitate to pick up the phone for fear they're being over-sensitive or a hypochondriac. While a good dose of common sense should be used in contacting your doctor after hours (for example, a call regarding the pros and cons of epidurals is probably not a good idea at 3 A.M.—unless you're in labor, of course), in most cases "better safe than sorry" applies. Remember, your provider works for you, and you're heading up this pregnancy team. Learn to trust your instincts. If something just doesn't feel right to you, make the call.

On Your Mind

Pregnancy, particularly a first pregnancy, is a time of great anticipation as you head into uncharted waters. Now that you've been to your first prenatal appointment and have officially started this journey, you may be surprised to find yourself filled with conflicting emotions.

Elation and Excitement

If this is a planned pregnancy, particularly a hard-earned one, you may be thrilled beyond belief. Of course, even the little surprises can be sources of great joy. You are creating a new and unique life of boundless potential. As a family, you will share your hopes, dreams, knowledge, and love. This is one of the most important tasks—and special experiences—of your life. So, excitement and even a few high-fives are the order of the day.

Anxiety

Worries about the baby's health and the possibility of miscarriage are common fears early in pregnancy. If you've had a previous miscarriage, you may be walking on eggshells trying to second-guess every move you make. The good news is that knowing your history of miscarriage, your provider is following your progress closely.

Although easier said than done, letting go of your anxieties, at least for a little while, is the best thing for you and your baby right now. Try designating a certain area of your home, like your bedroom, a worry-free zone, and then stick to a vow to let your anxieties go when you are in that space. Use sounds, sights, and smells to make it as comfortable and relaxing as possible. An aromatherapy candle that you like, soft music or nature sounds, and some soothing scenery in the form of photographs and posters can do wonders for your state of mind.

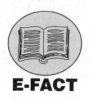

E-FACT

Feeling drippy? Pregnancy hormones may have you producing excess saliva, a condition called *ptyalism*. Postnasal drip or nasal congestion is another common side effect of hormonal changes. Both of these may be at least partial contributors to an unsettled stomach or morning sickness.

You might also be concerned about your ability to provide for and care for your child. It's important to remember that good parents learn with experience and by the experiences of others. The very fact that you're reading this book and getting regular prenatal care shows that you want the best for your baby. By the time your little bundle arrives, you'll be surprised at how much you will have learned in the relatively short period of 9 months.

Morning Sickness

Your stomach flutters, then lurches. As your mouth starts to water, you run for the bathroom for the fifth time today. Sound familiar? Morning sickness (NVP) is arguably the most debilitating and prevalent of pregnancy symptoms. While most women find that NVP symptoms subside or stop as the first trimester ends, for some they continue into the second and even third trimesters. If you're having twins or more, your NVP may be longer and more intense.

E-QUESTION

I can't stand wearing perfume anymore! Can pregnancy cause my nose to go haywire?

Pregnancy causes a heightened sensitivity to certain odors—coffee, cigarette smoke, and fried foods are frequent offenders—that can contribute to stomach unrest. One theory is that these olfactory aversions are your body's way of keeping you away from substances that could harm your developing baby.

The exact cause of NVP has not been pinpointed, but theories abound. Some possible culprits: the human chorionic gonadotropin (hCG) hormone that surges through your system and peaks in early pregnancy; a deficiency of vitamin B_6; hormonal changes that relax your gastrointestinal tract and slow digestion; and immune system changes. Another hypothesis is that morning sickness is actually a defense mechanism that protects both mother and child from toxins and potentially harmful microorganisms in food. No matter what the trigger, it's a miserable time for all.

Remedies and Safety

The following treatments have met with some success in lessening symptoms of NVP in clinical trials. (Speak with your health care provider before adding any new supplements to your diet.)

- **Ginger.** Gingersnaps and other foods and teas that contain ginger (*Zingiber officinale*) may be helpful in settling your stomach.

- **Acupressure wristbands (Sea-Bands).** Sometimes used to ward off motion sickness and seasickness, these wristbands place pressure on what is called the P6, or Nei-Kuan, acupressure point. Available at most drugstores, they are an inexpensive and noninvasive way to treat NVP.

- **Vitamin B$_6$.** This supplement has reduced NVP symptoms in several clinical trials. It has been suggested that NVP is a sign of B$_6$ vitamin deficiency.

E-ALERT!

> Kava-kava (*Piper methysticum*), licorice root (*Glycyrrhiza glabra*), rue (*Ruta graveolens*), Chinese cinnamon (*Cinnamomum aromaticum*), and safflower (*Carthamus tinctorius*, false saffron) are just a few of the many botanical remedies that are known to be dangerous in pregnancy. Don't pick up that supplement or cup of herbal tea without asking your health care provider first.

Other treatments that women report as helpful include:

✓ **Eating smaller, more frequent meals.** An empty stomach produces acid that can make you feel worse. Low blood sugar causes nausea as well.

✓ **Choosing proteins and complex carbohydrates.** Protein-rich foods (for example, yogurt, beans) and complex carbs (for example, baked potato, whole-grain breads) are good for the two of you and may calm your stomach.

✓ **Eat what you like.** Most pregnant women have at least one food aversion. If broccoli turns your tummy, don't force it. The better foods look and taste, the more likely they are to stay down.

✓ **Drink plenty of fluids.** Don't get dehydrated. If you're vomiting, you need to replace those lost fluids. Some women report better tolerance of beverages if they are taken between meals rather than with them.

Turned off by water and juice right now? Try juicy fruits like watermelon and grapes instead.

✓ **Brush regularly.** Keeping your mouth fresh can cut down on the excess saliva that plagues some pregnant women. Breath mints may be helpful, too.

✓ **Talk to your provider about switching prenatal supplements.** If it makes you sick just to look at your vitamins, perhaps a chewable or other formulation will help. Iron is notoriously tough on the stomach, so your provider might also recommend a supplement with a lower or extended-release dose. And if you can't keep your vitamins down no matter what you try, your doctor may suggest foregoing them until your NVP has passed.

How to Cope

Constant queasiness and vomiting may have you wondering why on earth you got pregnant in the first place. Try to take solace in the fact that for most women, NVP is primarily a first-trimester affair. Stick close to home and take it easy, if at all possible. When staying home isn't an option, talk to your employer about allowing some flexibility with your work schedule. If your stomach is at its worst first thing in the morning, ask about starting later in the day on a temporary basis. Depending on your occupation, working from home on some days may be an option.

When It May Be More Than Morning Sickness

When your body can't get what it needs from food to keep things running, it will start to metabolize stored fat for energy. This condition, called *ketosis*, generates *ketones* that circulate in your bloodstream and can be harmful to your fetus. Your provider may test your urine for ketones if you're having severe and persistent nausea and vomiting.

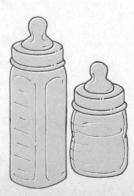

A small percentage of pregnant women (0.3 to 3 percent) experience a severe form of morning sickness called *hyperemesis gravidarum* (excessive vomiting of pregnancy). If you can't keep any food or fluids down, are losing weight, and are finding it impossible to function normally, you may be in this category.

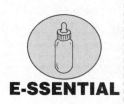

E-SSENTIAL

Put together a morning sickness survival kit for the car. Items to include: wet wipes, tissues, small bottle of water, travel-sized tooth-brush and toothpaste, breath mints, graham or soda crackers, and a bundle of large freezer-grade zip-top baggies (for obvious reasons!). For longer trips, a cell phone and a just-in-case change of clothes are necessities.

Even though hospitalization is sometimes required for hyperemesis gravidarum, the good news is that the treatment—intravenous fluids to restore fluid and electrolyte balance and, in some cases, antiemetics (drugs to stop vomiting)—is relatively simple. If you are prescribed antiemetics, talk with your doctor about the safety data for the drug prescribed and any potential effects on the fetus.

Just for Dads

Fathers have their own unique roles in pregnancy. Even though you are not physically carrying this child (likely a source of enormous relief as you watch your partner struggle with morning sickness and other pregnancy fun), you are sharing the emotional weight of pregnancy and experiencing the same fears, joys, and occasional bewilderment as your significant other. In many cases, you also have the added responsibility of being her primary source of support. In fact, this may be the first time in your lives when she is in charge of the manual labor and you're the emotional caregiver. Try to enjoy this new vantage point: Think of it as training for life as a dad.

This Wild Ride Called *Pregnancy*

Although your partner might not look very pregnant yet, chances are she's acting like it. Mood swings (emotional lability, in medical terminology) are the result of the many hormonal changes pregnancy brings and may be one of the first things you notice. So, if you're laughing together one minute and being yelled at the next, don't take it personally. It's all part of the package.

Morning sickness, particularly when it is severe, can be a disturbing part of pregnancy for men. Supporting your partner during this difficult time—making sure she gets adequate rest, taking care of household duties, and catering to her food requests, no matter how odd they may seem—is the best way you can help both her and your child.

Fear of the Future

It's natural to feel rattled about providing for an utterly dependent and so tiny a person. Practical matters, like being able to support a bigger family, may be dominating your thoughts right now. If you haven't already, talk with your spouse or partner about your concerns; chances are she shares many of the same anxieties you do, and working together as a family is the best way to face them head-on.

Family Matters

No matter what shape and size your current household, the arrival of a new baby in your home will touch your life in ways you never imagined. Just about every aspect of your daily routine is going to change—how you eat, sleep, play, and work. As you wait to welcome your child into the world, take advantage of this time to lay the foundation for your expanding family circle.

Make Room for Baby

Kids are remarkably adaptable. They can thrive in just about any location, given a healthy and nurturing environment. They do need a safe space to grow in, however; babies learn through exploring and experiencing their immediate surroundings.

A Space of Her Own

Start thinking about where your baby will be sleeping and playing so that you can coordinate logistics and gear. Keep an open mind as to arrangements, however. Even if you can't wait to see your little angel peacefully dozing against his color-coordinated crib sheets, you might have second thoughts about having him all the way down the hall once he arrives (especially when the 2 A.M. feeding rolls around).

Some parents choose to keep their newborns in their bedrooms, either in a crib or bassinet or in the parental bed—a somewhat controversial practice known as *co-sleeping*. Proponents of co-sleeping say that it encourages breastfeeding, boosts mom's milk production, and provides a better bonding experience for parents and baby. Critics cite studies finding that bed sharing disrupts sleep patterns and increases the risk of SIDS. However, factors such as baby's sleep position, type of bedding, and parental smoking and alcohol consumption raise SIDS risk as well, and it isn't completely clear whether bed sharing in the absence of these risk factors still presents a significant hazard.

E-FACT

The American Association of Pediatrics advises in their latest policy statement that to reduce the risk of SIDS, "a separate but proximate sleeping environment is recommended." So the baby should sleep in the same room as mom but the AAP suggests that the baby sleep in a crib, bassinet, or cradle.

Whatever you decide regarding your baby's sleeping arrangements (and you may not decide until you actually have her in your arms), if you have the space you're probably already laying plans for the baby's room. If you're torn about giving up your study for a nursery (after all, she'll be small; how much space can she need?), think about the baby basics (crib, changing area, dresser) plus all the inevitable stuff you're bound to acquire—swings, stuffed animals, bouncy chairs, baby books, bathtubs—and the choice becomes clear.

If a nursery isn't an option due to the size of your home, there are several ways to give baby a place of her own. A folding screen (or two) or curtains hung from a ceiling track can be a creative way to close off part of a room. If you have the money but limited room, think of building out a wall for a more permanent partition.

E-ALERT!

Make sure baby sleeps safely on a firm mattress, without soft bedding or duvets. Always place him on his back to sleep, and never share a bed with a baby after you have been drinking or if you are under the influence of drugs that alter consciousness.

Wherever it is, the baby's space should be well-ventilated and insulated. Evaluate the area for safety hazards such as peeling paint, dangling blind cords, and loose flooring. If there are door stoppers installed, make sure they are one piece; the rubber bumper on many models presents a choking hazard. When it comes time to purchase a crib, make sure it has no decorative features that could potentially catch on clothing or entrap the baby, and that the crib slats are a maximum of 2⅜ inches apart. The crib should also meet the latest safety standards and not have drop-down side rails. The mattress should fit snugly against the crib sides.

Bye Bye Miata, Hello Minivan

Time to face the cold, hard facts: that sporty two-seater just isn't going to hack it once you have both a baby and all her associated cargo to carry about town. Cast a critical eye toward your current vehicle, and make sure it meets both the practical and safety concerns of your growing family. Some things to look for:

✓ **Sit back and be safe.** The best place for any child is in the back seat. If you have the choice, avoid pickup trucks or other vehicles that don't offer one.

✓ **Preferred seating.** Size matters, and so does shape. Make sure baby's car seat fits properly in the vehicle and there is adequate room if you have more than one child to secure.

✓ **Passenger airbag on/off switch.** If your new baby must ride in the front passenger seat and there is an airbag, there absolutely *must* be a switch that allows you to disengage the airbag on that side. Permission to install a switch can be obtained from the National Highway Traffic Safety Administration (NHTSA). Check with your state motor vehicle bureau for details.

✓ **Study the side airbag.** Rear-seat side-impact airbags (SABs) at the chest and head/chest levels can also pose a significant risk of injury to children, while roof-mounted head SABs are considered safe. If the vehicle has an activated rear-seat side airbag, check with the car manufacturer or the NHTSA to make sure it has been adequately tested for safe use with children. Otherwise, have it deactivated.

✓ **Locking seat belts, tethers, or anchors.** Most vehicles built after 2002 accommodate a LATCH system (lower anchors and tethers for children) that allows you to secure the top and side tethers on a LATCH-equipped child seat to anchors built into the car's interior. If your car seat or vehicle is not LATCH-equipped, cars built after 1996 should have seat belts that work with most car seats. Always check the owner's manual of your vehicle and car seat for proper installation instructions.

✓ **Interior trunk release.** If your car was manufactured after September 2001, it should have a release mechanism inside the trunk to prevent curious children from becoming trapped inside. Retrofitted release latches are available for cars without this feature.

✓ **Don't run hot and cold.** If your car's heating and cooling system is out of commission, now is the time to get it fixed. An infant's internal thermostat is not as efficient as an adult's, and your child can quickly become overheated or chilled.

✓ **Accessorize.** Car seat belts and buckles left in the sun can pose a burn hazard to infants. Consider a car seat cover or window and windshield sun screens, which are useful in preventing your car's interior from absorbing the sun's heat.

Other features that may be helpful but aren't essential include built-in child car seats, safety door locks, rearview cameras, a blind spot assist system, and collision mitigation braking systems.

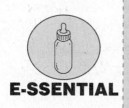

E-SSENTIAL

Airbags can save lives, but when used improperly, they can also cause serious injuries. A rear-facing infant seat in the front passenger seat places your child's head just inches from the airbag, which deploys with tremendous force and speed—a potentially fatal combination. All kids under thirteen should buckle up in the back seat whenever possible.

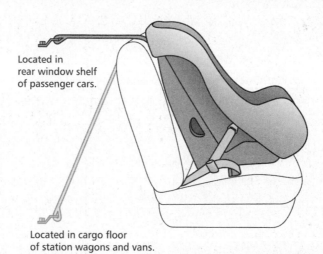

Located in rear window shelf of passenger cars.

Located in cargo floor of station wagons and vans.

The LATCH system—Lower Anchors and Tethers for Children—uses anchors mounted in the seat cushion and a top tether to secure a child safety seat

Babyproof

Now that you have car safety covered, take a look at potential hazards inside your home. Although your home safety efforts will undoubtedly pick up steam as your child gets mobile and starts exploring her surroundings, there are some basic things you can do now to protect her in infancy and beyond.

✓ **Register for recalls.** Take the time to fill out those registration cards for all the baby gear you receive. If a safety recall of the product occurs, the manufacturer will be able to notify you. You can also register for e-mail alerts of new product recalls from the U.S. Consumer Product Safety Commission at *www.cpsc.gov.*

✓ **Ban cigarettes.** You already know how dangerous it is to smoke during pregnancy, but did you know that secondhand smoke, particularly in a closed home environment, is harmful to your baby's health? Tobacco is also toxic when eaten; because babies put just about everything in their mouths, that's just one more good reason to make your home a tobacco-free zone.

✓ **Get the lead out.** Lead paint, most frequently found in homes built before 1978, is a major hazard to small children. When ingested, either by eating paint chips or breathing in lead dust, it can cause central nervous system (CNS) damage and a host of other health and developmental problems. Lead solder used in some older plumbing systems can also pose a risk. If you haven't done so already, contact a lead inspector certified by the state and/or the U.S. Environmental Protection Agency (EPA) to test your home for the presence of lead and to advise you on abatement procedures, if necessary. And be sure to test for lead paint prior to any renovations or construction. If lead is present, you may have to live somewhere else until the dust clears.

✓ **Rearrange the furniture.** Block off electrical cords and buy plastic protectors to seal open outlets. Pad sharp table corners to protect baby from injury. Evaluate your home from a baby's eye view (about

3 feet off the floor, for good measure), and move anything dangerous, expensive, or breakable to higher ground.

✓ **Practice.** Some old habits—like leaving the toilet seat up—are hard to break. It will be easy to be vigilant later if you get accustomed to baby-safe behavior now. A few new routines to try out: store medications, cleaning products, and other toxic substances out of a child's reach; store plastic bags in a latched cabinet; make sure all members of the household leave the toilet seat and lid down; set your hot water heater to 120°F; install carbon monoxide detector, and test your smoke alarms.

The High Cost of Having a Baby

If you have substantial or full insurance coverage for your prenatal care and delivery expenses, you can breathe a sigh of relief. According to an Agency for Heatlhcare Research and Quality report released in 2010, average hospital charges for delivering a baby in 2008 were $3,400 for an uncomplicated delivery and $5,700 for an uncomplicated cesarean section. Average cost climbs to $9,400 for a vaginal delivery with an operating procedure. And prenatal care adds another several thousand to the bill; however, studies show that such expenses are more than offset by improved outcomes for both mother and child.

Insurance Issues

Review your insurance plan so that you are clear on the extent and nature of your coverage for both prenatal care and labor and delivery. If you have questions, call your insurance company or speak to the benefits coordinator at your workplace.

Keep on top of insurance problems. As any physician's or hospital's billing department can tell you, insurance companies do occasionally lose and mishandle claims. Whenever you call either your provider's billing department or the insurance company, take notes summarizing the conversation, including a date to follow up, and the name of the person you speak with. If you're trying to unravel a knotty insurance issue, being able to track it with someone who is familiar with your case will save you time and aggravation. And if you aren't getting action, it helps to document exactly who has dropped the ball as you move up the chain of command. Follow up with letters and request written documentation of any actions taken over the phone so that you have a paper trail as well.

Payment Options

If you have a large deductible to pay out of pocket, or are responsible for a hefty percentage of your physician's bill, don't panic. Work with your provider's office to negotiate a realistic payment schedule. Contact the business office of the hospital or birthing center where you will deliver for registration information and details on their billing terms. Some providers and hospitals may have maternity assistance programs, including sliding fee scales and prepayment discounts.

Ways to Save

According to U.S. Census Bureau estimates, 16.7 percent of all Americans were without health insurance in 2009. There are public aid programs available if you are uninsured and unable to meet the financial obligations of prenatal care and childbirth.

Medicaid is a state-run public assistance program that provides medical care to low-income families at little to no cost. For information on qualifying standards, see the federal Centers for Medicare and Medicaid Services' website at *www.cms.gov* or call your state social services department.

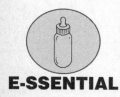

E-SSENTIAL

Make sure you find out the procedure for putting the newest member of your family on your insurance policy once he arrives. If you're paying insurance premiums, find out what the additional charge will be so that you can budget for it now.

The Special Supplemental Nutrition Program for Women, Infants, and Children (WIC) is a federally funded, state-administered program targeted to nutritionally at-risk women (both pregnant and postpartum) and children up to age 5. WIC provides food vouchers to those who meet qualifying guidelines and have an annual gross household income that does not exceed 185 percent of the federal poverty level ($41,348 for a family of four in the forty-eight contiguous states in 2011; slightly higher in Alaska and Hawaii).

The Children's Health Insurance Program (CHIP) is a federal program that covers infants and children in families that are financially strained but earn income levels too high to qualify for Medicaid. If you're concerned about insurance coverage for your newborn, call 1-877-KIDS-NOW or visit *www.insurekidsnow.gov* for more details.

There may be other financial assistance available in your area. Contact your area social services agency for more details.

Bargain Hunters

Even if you've never been one to clip coupons, the expense of keeping baby in diapers and other essentials is a strong incentive to start looking for savings. Next time you're at the doctor's office, take a look around the waiting room for product offers. Many new-parent clubs have cropped up, supported by formula makers, diaper manufacturers, and other baby product companies, and they often recruit members right there at the source.

Some kid-focused retailers also have coupon clubs. Sign up if you'd like to receive free product samples and coupons. One caveat: putting your name on their mailing lists may open you up to a deluge of junk mail from so-called "valued partners." Check out the form you sign for its printed privacy policy if this is a concern; it may offer you an opportunity to opt out of such mailings.

There are several free magazines on the market geared specifically for new parents and moms-to-be, again often available right at your provider's office. Be aware that because the publishers make their money from advertisers rather than from subscribers, these publications are typically laden with product ads. However, they still have lots of useful new parenting information and an abundance of coupons and free offers.

Check your local library for other community or regional parenting publications that can point you toward useful family resources and, again, those handy coupons.

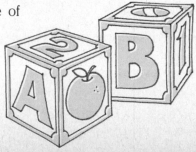

Although breastmilk is the least expensive way to feed your baby (along with its many other extraordinary health benefits), if you are planning on bottle-feeding, freebies abound. Formula is expensive, and baby will eventually be putting away about 30 ounces a day (900 ounces per month). Acquiring a loyal customer through free samples and other incentives makes good business sense to formula manufacturers, who are big on the aforementioned new-parent clubs. They also provide a steady stream of samples to prenatal care providers and pediatricians. If you don't see samples or aren't offered any, ask your provider.

Finally, if you deliver in a hospital, make sure you get what you pay for. Chances are you'll be billed for all the items you and your newborn use—including the pacifier, nasal aspirator, sanitary napkins, alcohol swabs, open bags of diapers and wipe cloths, and even the little plastic comb for baby's hair (whether baby has any or not). By all means, take these with you when you leave! Ask the nurse what is fair game. Often the hospital staff can send you home with even more free product samples than you will find in your hospital room.

Financial Planning for a Bigger Family

Hold on to your hats. According to the U.S. Department of Agriculture (USDA), a child born in 2010 costs the average parents between $226,920 and $377,040 (depending on income level) by the time she reaches age 17. If you've been living an unbudgeted lifestyle, now is a good time to start setting up a family spending and savings plan.

Cost Comparisons

Clueless about baby care costs? Take a reconnaissance mission to the grocery store to gather prices on diapers, wipes, and other essentials. If you're considering day care or an in-home babysitter, now is also a good time to get information and monthly cost estimates. As usual, other parents are an excellent source of tips and leads to the best resources in your area.

E-FACT

In 1 week, the average baby goes through about sixty to eighty diaper changes. That's a potential pile up of 4,160 diapers in the first year alone! If you're using disposable ones, price out cases of diapers at the local warehouse club or discount store because bulk purchases are typically cheaper.

Don't forget to factor in pediatric care and additional health insurance premiums on your bottom line. If you belong to an HMO or other managed-care health plan, it's probable that well-baby visits are covered at 100 percent or with a minimal copay. You may want to review your health insurance options now so that when baby comes you can enroll her in the most appropriate and cost-effective program.

Setting Savings Goals

Now that you've figured out what you'll be spending on baby care, of what practical use is this? Lay out your current spending habits, including basic monthly bills like utilities and housing, debts that can be downsized (for example, credit cards and car payments), transportation costs, food and household goods, health care, and discretionary/disposable income. Accounting for everything in black and white will give you a much clearer picture of where you're spending and the size of any gap between income and expenses. This can also help you figure out big-picture questions like whether you have the financial means to switch to a part-time schedule at work.

When it comes time to balance your home budget, be realistic in your planning and prudent when you eliminate discretionary purchases; brown-bagging it to work each and every day for the next 3 years is a noble goal, but a weekly or biweekly meal out with colleagues could pay off in other ways. Give yourself a little breathing room for unforeseen emergency expenses like an appliance meltdown or car repairs. A little scrimping here, one less latte a week there, and you'll find budgeting easier than you thought.

Some parents find it daunting to consider long-term expenses, like college, when the costs and responsibilities of child rearing itself seem so overwhelming. Just remember that early planning can net big returns over time. If you start saving just $50 a month in a savings account or other interest-bearing investment at a 5 percent interest rate when your child is born, you will have $16,026 by the time your child is ready to start college. If you don't know an IRA from the NRA, you might want to sit down with a financial advisor to discuss college savings options. She might also be able to assist you in re-evaluating your life insurance needs, something else that should be done periodically as your family grows.

Lifestyle Changes, or Stating the Obvious

Your baby's arrival will transform just about everything you think, say, and do. This sea change is usually most evident with first-time parents, who up until now have been enjoying the child-free pursuits of quiet dinners, R-rated movies, and even the occasional wild night out with the girls or boys. Even those moms and dads who are expecting a second or subsequent child will have big adjustments ahead with new challenges like siblinghood and advanced parental multitasking (for example, encouraging one child to use his napkin while preventing the other from eating hers). Don't look on it as an end but rather as a new and infinitely more rewarding chapter in your life. You will even find some family pastimes you have never considered before.

Sharing Pregnancy with the Dad-to-Be

With the big focus on mom and her growing belly, it's easy for dads to get overlooked in the pregnancy drama. Remind your significant other that you're in this together. If he isn't quite sure of his role in this new adventure yet, he could be looking to you for cues. Encourage him to join you at prenatal checkups as well as share pregnancy education and experiences like the first kicks. You should also try to pencil in some special couple time to talk to baby, contemplate names, and share your hopes and dreams about your family's future.

From Two to Three

The new person in your life has already started competing for your attention, changing your eating and sleeping patterns, and perhaps slowing down your pace. Unexpected emotions may surface between you and your significant other as your pregnancy progresses. He may feel pangs of jealousy at the loss of your couplehood and your focus on the baby. On the flip side, you may be feeling as if you're playing second fiddle to your future child as the prospective father questions the safety of every move you make. Such growing pains are normal. Try to talk about your feelings and approach parenting (even now) as a team effort.

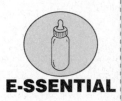

E-SSENTIAL

Strange but true: men can have pregnancy symptoms, too. Known as *couvade syndrome*, this sympathy-pain phenomenon may have your significant other experiencing nausea, fatigue, weight gain, and mood swings. What's behind it? Anxiety associated with impending fatherhood is suspected by some, but one Canadian study found that men experiencing couvade symdrome had distinct hormonal changes that mirrored their pregnant partners.

Some dads are intimidated by the size and vulnerability of an infant and as a result pass on most of the child care responsibilities to the mother, a potential lose-lose situation for both of you. If he is feeling uneasy about his lack of experience in the child care arena, suggest a few tag-team babysitting sessions for a niece or nephew or a friend's child to build his confidence.

The Bond of Parenthood

Pregnancy can bring a couple closer together than they ever imagined, but it can also present new frictions in your relationship. The aches and pains of pregnancy can push the most even-tempered woman to her limits. Add to that a healthy surge of estrogen and progesterone, and you have the recipe for major mood swings. Other stressors, like a tepid sex life and financial fears, can also stir the pot. Try to approach these temporary changes with understanding and empathy for your partner and a healthy sense of humor, if at all possible.

Single Moms and Support

If you're a single mother-to-be by choice or by circumstance, you aren't alone. Well over a third of all women (41 percent) who gave birth in 2009 were unmarried, according to the U.S. Centers for Disease Control and Prevention. Pregnancy and birth are physically and emotionally challenging experiences. As a single mom, you may also have the added baggage of financial, career, and custody concerns weighing on you. Dealing positively with the stress is important for both your own health and that of your baby.

E-QUESTION

I'm single, a college student, and pregnant. Where can I turn for financial help?
Some student health insurance programs cover prenatal care and delivery costs, and many schools offer day care facilities that can help you continue your studies once your baby arrives. Check with your university counseling center for more information. You may also qualify for public aid programs like WIC.

Don't fly solo if you don't have to. Enlist a family member or a close friend to accompany you on prenatal visits, to childbirth classes, and during the birth itself. A doula can also be a wonderful source of support for labor and delivery. If possible, make arrangements for a live-in companion for the first few postpartum weeks as well.

An Eye Toward the Future

They may seem worlds away now, but matters like schools, parks, and playgroups are waiting just around the corner. As you talk to other parents and families in your neighborhood, start to gather information on the resources available in your area. If you are hunting for a bigger home in anticipation of your new arrival, be sure to investigate the school district possibilities and community resources now to save yourself another move in 5 years.

Kids in Community

That oft-said proverb "It takes a whole village to raise a child" is true. The community in which you raise your child will play a large part in shaping her values, beliefs, and personality. You will be the gatekeeper for her early exposure to the outside world, of course, but schools, playgroups, and community services that reinforce your value system will make parenting your growing child a group effort rather than a solitary endeavor. Just as important will be your own personal investment in these institutions as you give of your time and talents.

It's not too early to get involved with a playgroup when your baby is just a few months old, as he will enjoy playing with you and observing other kids in a group setting. Investigate what's already available in your area, or talk to some parents and moms-to-be in your neighborhood about starting up something new once the baby arrives. Laying the foundation now for friendships and positive community relationships will help your child flourish.

Faith and Family

New parents often find themselves exploring their roots and reconnecting with their own childhoods. Even if your extended family lives far away, you can still share the special moments of your pregnancy and birth through photos, videotapes, and phone calls. Sharing the parenting experience across generations can be a powerful experience that forges a special bond with grandparents. And when Thanksgiving comes, you'll finally feel like you belong at the adult table.

Before you became pregnant, spirituality may have taken a back seat in your busy life. Now that you are going to have a child to raise and educate, the traditions and values of your faith, whatever it is, are going to take on a new dimension. If you and your partner come from different religious backgrounds, this subject holds special significance. Will you choose one organized religion over the other or expose your child to both faiths? If you're concerned about baptism, an interfaith service that respects the traditions and beliefs of two-religion families is an option. It is important to open up family communication by talking about your expectations now.

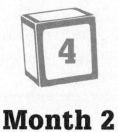

Month 2

You've made it into month 2, or weeks 6 through 10, of your pregnancy. By the end of this month, your baby will outgrow its embryonic development and mature into a fetus. Your body is changing rapidly; you may start to feel pregnant now, if you didn't feel so before.

Baby This Month

Your unborn child has now advanced from raisin to raspberry size—about a half inch in length. By the end of the month, she will be about an inch long (like a good-sized grape). The fetus is lengthening and straightening from the shrimplike, curled form it held last month. The tail she was sporting disappears around week 8, and her closed eyes start to move from the sides of the head to their permanent location. The face is further defined by a nose and jaw, and the buds of twenty tiny baby teeth are present in the gums by week 10. The palate and vocal cords also form around this time, although baby isn't ready to make herself heard just yet.

Important organ systems are nearly completed by the end of this 2nd month. The right and left hemispheres of your baby's brain are fully formed, and brain cell mass grows rapidly. Soft bones begin to develop, and the liver starts to manufacture red blood cells until the bone marrow can take over the job in the third trimester.

E-FACT

Boy or girl? Although external sex organs begin to differentiate this month, they won't become visible on an ultrasound until around weeks 16 to 20. If you're scheduled for an amniocentesis, the gender of your child can be definitively determined at that time. Then again, you might enjoy the element of surprise by waiting until birth to find out your baby's gender.

Your unborn baby is also giving his brand new organs a workout. Heart chambers form, the pancreas begins to produce insulin, and the liver secretes bile. The stomach produces gastric juices, while the intestines, which have developed in the umbilical cord, move up into the abdomen by the end of the month.

Floating in about 1.5 ounces (approximately 10 teaspoons) of amniotic fluid, your baby has plenty of room for flexing the muscles she is now developing. Because of her small size and spacious accommodations, chances are you won't notice these movements now. At about weeks 18 to 20, when the second trimester is in full swing and her quarters become a bit closer, you will feel the first flutterings, known as *quickening*.

E-ALERT!

If you are at risk for passing on a hereditary health condition to your child, you may choose to schedule a chorionic villus sampling (CVS) at the end of this month. A CVS is typically administered between weeks 10 and 12 and involves taking a small sample of placental tissue for laboratory analysis.

Your Body This Month

If you weren't feeling very pregnant last month, you are probably starting to now. About midway through this month, hCG levels will begin to peak and then slowly decline as the placenta starts to produce the pregnancy hormones progesterone and estradiol. The ebb and flow of your hormones will trigger a few new pregnancy symptoms this month.

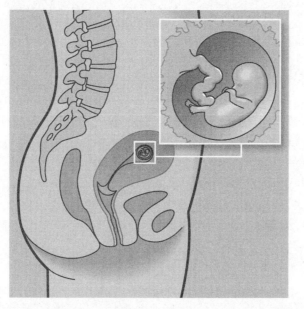

At the end of month 2, your baby is officially a fetus

Your Body Changes

Even though you may not have put on any additional weight yet, your growing uterus is pushing the boundaries of your waistline. On average, most women gain 2 to 4 pounds in the first trimester.

Changes in skin and hair are common in pregnancy. Hair that was fine and thin may become thick and shiny during pregnancy, and that fabled pregnancy glow may actually be your flawless, blemish-free complexion. On the other end of the spectrum, acne problems and hair breakage and thinning may occur.

Chloasma (also known as *melasma*) may cause a mask-like darkening or lightening of your facial skin. Freckles and moles are prone to darkening as are other pigmented areas of your skin (for example, areolae). To minimize chloasma and other hyperpigmentation, use a good sunscreen (SPF 30 or higher) to cover exposed skin when you're out in the sun.

E-QUESTION

Will coloring my hair hurt my baby?
To date, there is no conclusive evidence that hair-color use in pregnancy is dangerous. If you are concerned over a possible risk, you may opt for a vegetable-based or temporary color treatment until the baby is born. Some experts also recommend holding off on all chemical hair treatments during the first trimester.

Your gums may start to bleed when you brush your teeth, a condition known as *pregnancy gingivitis*. Be sure to floss and brush regularly to keep your teeth and gums healthy. A warm saltwater rinse may soothe swollen gum tissues. Now is a good time to schedule a thorough cleaning with your dentist; in a few months, leaning back in a dental chair will be uncomfortable, if not impossible. Gum disease has been associated with preterm labor, so keep up with regular dental checkups during pregnancy.

What You Feel Like

The stomach rumblings of the first month continue, and an increase in nausea and vomiting may actually occur as hCG levels peak toward the end of this month. On the plus side, your NVP may start to get better in the coming weeks as hCG levels wane. If you're one of those lucky women who do not experience morning sickness at all, you're probably not escaping the feelings of fatigue. Take the hint your body is giving you to take time out to rest.

Other symptoms that may start or continue this month include:

✓ Frequent urination
✓ Tender, larger breasts
✓ Increased vaginal discharge
✓ Occasional dizziness or faintness
✓ Indigestion or gas
✓ Headaches
✓ Nasal congestion and/or runny nose
✓ Increased saliva

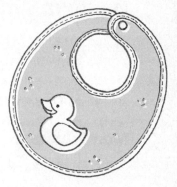

At Your Doctor Visit

If you had your preliminary appointment last month, your prenatal office visits will now start to slip into a routine. At a minimum, expect to step on the scale, give a urine sample, and have your blood pressure checked at the start of each appointment. You'll also be asked about any new or continuing pregnancy symptoms, and your provider will feel the outside of your abdomen to determine the size of your uterus.

Get the Most Out of Monthly Checkups

Bring along that list of questions that have come up since your last visit. Again, write these down when they come to you and your partner so that you won't have to rely on your memory in the doctor's office. And make sure your questions are answered before you leave; although it's nice to be asked if you have any concerns, in the busy atmosphere of an obstetric practice your provider may occasionally forget. Stop her before she leaves the exam room, and let her know that you have a few questions. Never feel like you're being pushy or overbearing (remember, you're leading this team). In most cases she will do what she can to educate you and reduce any anxieties. If she doesn't, it's never too late to find someone who will.

Tests This Month

Additional blood tests for Rhesus (Rh) factor and rubella antibodies may be ordered this month if they were not taken at your last appointment.

On Your Mind

Now that you're feeling more symptoms of pregnancy, the reality of impending parenthood may suddenly hit home. "So much to do, so little time," you may be thinking. Understanding and recognizing your emotional changes can help you better control your stress levels.

Mood Swings

Find yourself laughing hysterically or sobbing uncontrollably? If you're normally the even-keeled type, these emotional outbursts can be downright alarming. You aren't losing control or losing your mind; you're just experiencing the normal mood swings of pregnancy. Although this emotional roller coaster may continue throughout pregnancy, it is typically strongest in the first trimester as you adjust to hormonal and other changes.

E-ALERT!

If you have a cat, try to hand over litter box duties to someone else. Toxoplasmosis, a parasitical infection passed on by infected cat feces (also by undercooked meat and infected unwashed raw vegetables), has the potential to cause brain damage and other medical problems in your unborn child. Cats also frequent gardens and sandboxes, so wear gloves, and wash your hands thoroughly after working outside.

Given the transformation your body is going through and the accompanying aches and pains, you have every right to be cranky. In fact, when you factor in your physical discomforts with the spectrum of emotions you're experiencing as motherhood approaches, you've got a license to be hell on wheels. Of course, no one is happy when that happens (just ask your partner), so take steps now to reduce your stress level and achieve some balance.

Stress and Stress Management

It's easy to get stressed out over what may seem like an overwhelming amount of preparation for your new family member. Your body is already working overtime on the development of your child; try to keep your commitments and activities at a reasonable level to prevent mental and physical overload.

Controlling outer stress is especially important when your pregnant body is under the physical stress of providing for a growing baby. And added psychological stress can make the discomforts of pregnancy last longer and feel more severe.

E-FACT

Some traditional stress-control methods, such as relaxation techniques involving certain strenuous yoga positions or martial arts, are not appropriate for pregnant women. You should also not try fad diets, herbal preparations, or over-the-counter medications (which are generally not good stress control methods, in any case). When in doubt, check with your health care provider.

Anxiety may also impact your unborn child's health. An increase of corticotropin-releasing hormone (CRH), a stress-related substance produced by the brain and the placenta, has been linked to preterm labor and low birth weight. Research has also suggested a possible connection between first-trimester maternal stress and congenital malformations.

As you rush to get everything just so, remember that your little one is not going to care if the crib matches the dresser, but he will feel the effects of your excess tension. Keeping the ups and downs of pregnancy in perspective is important. So is taking steps to decompress when you feel the pressure building.

Effective stress management involves finding the right technique for you. Relaxation and meditation techniques (for example, progressive muscle relaxation, yoga), adjustments to your work or social schedule, or carving out an hour of "me time" each evening to decompress are all ways you can lighten your load. Exercise is also a great stress-control method, but be sure to get your doctor's approval regarding the level of exercise appropriate for you.

Dressing for Two

Finding maternity clothes that are fashionable, that fit, that grow comfortably with you, and that don't cost a fortune can be a challenge. Start out by deciding how much you want to spend; if you blow your whole clothing budget on a few items, you're going to be awfully limited in your wardrobe.

A few other things to keep in mind while you develop your wardrobe:

✓ **Consider your laundry threshold.** Check the tags to make sure that the care instructions mesh with your lifestyle. Hand washing your delicates may not top your priority list right now. And make sure you get enough maternity pieces so that you aren't washing the same three outfits constantly.

✓ **Mix and match.** Try to build on what you already own by adding pieces that will work well in a variety of combinations.

✓ **Keep your sense of style.** Although maternity clothes are getting more fashionable in response to women's needs, there are still plenty of overalls festooned with ruffles and appliqués, "I'm With Fetus" T-shirts, and similar maternity gear out there. Buy what you like; even if it takes a little searching, it will be worth it.

✓ **Built to last?** You'll only be wearing these clothes for a matter of months, so they don't need to be made to withstand a natural disaster. However, if you're planning on stretching their shelf life through another pregnancy, spending a little more on well-made, durable attire is more economical in the long run.

Look Good . . . Feel Good

Dressing well can improve your mood and self-image at a time when these may be shaky. Dressing well, according to your own personal style, does not necessarily mean dressing up. This could mean wearing a favorite jogging suit for running errands or a little (or big) black dress for a night out. Don't forget to purchase some nice loungewear or pajama sets for your take-it-easy days. Even when you're throwing up and miserable, slipping on something cozy can comfort your soul if not your stomach.

Shopping by Due Date

Think about the time of year when you'll be delivering, especially if you live in a region with a variable climate. Being 9 months pregnant in the dog days of summer and wearing the wool pants you bought midwinter will not be a good idea. To bridge the seasonal shifts, buy clothing that layers well—peeled down for summer and piled on for winter. Invest in mix-and-match pieces in breathable fabrics that are adaptable to temperature changes.

Beg, Borrow, and Rent

What could you possibly find in your partner's closet? Plenty, if you use a little imagination: oversize button-down oxfords and a fashion-forward Hawaiian shirt or two if you're feeling adventurous. Even some of his khakis or other casual slacks may be a good fit in the early months of pregnancy when you're too big for your old pants yet not quite at the maternity clothes stage. If you're just starting to show in late summer but want to save your clothing budget for fall and winter attire, borrow a pair or two of his cargo shorts to fill the gap.

If you and your significant other aren't a good size match, tap formerly pregnant friends and family for contributions. Take what you're offered—graciously. Even if the item doesn't look quite you at the outset, try matching it with some of your own pieces and accessorizing; the diversity may do your wardrobe some good. If it's beyond help, it can stay on the hanger and no one will be the wiser.

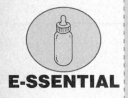

There is also a new breed of maternity clothing boutique, where for a monthly or weekly fee you can rent a selection of outfits to get you through pregnancy. The benefit is more variety in your wardrobe because you can switch out clothing on a regular basis. The downside is that if you're planning on a subsequent pregnancy, your investment won't leave you with anything to keep and wear again.

Dressed for Success

Women who work in an office or other professional environment have the added challenge and expense of finding appropriate clothes. Because of their limited lifespan in women's closets, maternity clothes make great resale shop fodder. Consignment stores that deal specifically in maternity wear are also becoming more commonplace. You may be surprised at some of the bargains you can uncover.

Just for Dads

Things get interesting this month as you both become familiar with the weird but wonderful world of the pregnant body. Step right up and witness the amazing expanding belly. Thrill to the fantastic swelling bust line! Dare to brave the snores and thrashes of the mother-to-be as she tries to find comfort in her natural sleeping habitat. This truly is the greatest show on earth.

Her Changing Body

Getting your libidos in sync during pregnancy can be a challenge. If she's experiencing nausea and vomiting right now, chances are she's not feeling too sexy. On the other hand, for some women the hormonal onslaught of pregnancy has their sexuality in overdrive. You too may feel a similar range of sensations and emotions as the pregnancy progresses. Although you may never have thought it possible, fears of somehow hurting the baby during intercourse and a new perception of your partner as a mother may have you shying away from the bedroom. Or you may find her physical metamorphosis, composure, and strength a highly sensual experience.

So, what do you do if you aren't on the same sexual wavelength? First of all, be sympathetic to the physical demands on her body right now, and remember that this is a temporary situation. She may be feeling insecure about her appearance or just awkward and clumsy as her body grows. Stress and anxiety can also douse her sex drive. Reassure her that she's still beautiful, perhaps even more so, and try to lighten her load by pitching in around the house and taking over some of the tasks that might be getting difficult for her (such as bending over to pick up your dirty socks).

If she's looking for love but you aren't, look at the reasons behind your feelings. Is safety a concern? Sex is safe and normal if the pregnancy is progressing normally. The baby is well-protected in the uterus. Be aware that an orgasm can sometimes trigger contractions, but these do not cause preterm labor in a normal, low-risk pregnancy.

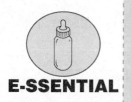

E-SSENTIAL

Most doctors advise pregnant women not to have sex if they are having preterm labor, premature cervical dilation, or complications from a placenta previa. Some physicians will also tell patients with a twin pregnancy, a history of incompetent cervix, or risk factors for premature delivery not to have intercourse.

If you're thinking "mommy" every time you see your wife and her baby bulge, you may have a harder time getting past your aversion to sexual intimacy. The most important thing is for you both to talk about it and discuss your feelings openly and honestly. Ignoring the problem will breed frustration and anger.

If you do agree to put sex on the back burner for a while, this doesn't mean a moratorium on romance. Bring her flowers, treat her to a weekend getaway, or just cook her dinner one night and spend the evening talking about the future. Above all, enjoy each other and keep your relationship healthy.

Sympathy Pains

Every day she seems to have a new and interesting pregnancy symptom to report. Suddenly you're feeling symptoms, too. Sympathetic pregnancy symptoms (couvade) are actually a fairly common occurrence. It's estimated that up to 65 percent of men experience one or more pregnancy symptoms during their partner's pregnancy, including nausea, backache, weight gain, and difficulty sleeping. The cause is likely multifaceted—a combination of psychological, social, and possibly even biological factors. They do say that misery loves company; take it as a signal to have some rest and recuperation time together.

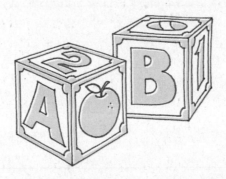

Diagnostic Tests and Screenings

As you likely suspect by now, you'll be poked, prodded, swabbed, scraped, and scanned throughout your pregnancy. All these tests have a purpose, of course—a healthy mom and baby. Prenatal tests elicit the full spectrum of maternal emotions, from calm reassurance (the staccato lub-dub of your baby's heart) to amusement (a fast fetal wave from the ultrasound screen) to anxiety and fear of the unknown. Knowing what to expect can make these exams more comfortable.

The Basics

At each visit to your provider, you'll have your blood pressure and weight checked and any swelling assessed. Overall, blood pressure tends to go down in pregnancy because of the increase in the size of the circulatory system, a more elastic cardiovascular system, and other factors. A normal blood pressure range in pregnancy is around 120 (systolic) over 70 (diastolic). Anything higher than 140 over 90 (written 140/90) is considered high. Your doctor will monitor any sudden elevations in blood pressure carefully, as they can be an early sign of pregnancy-induced hypertension or preeclampsia.

Your belly will be examined; just how depends on where you are in your pregnancy, but you might expect a regular measurement of your fundal height (the top of your uterus) starting sometime in the second trimester, and an external check of the baby's position in the third trimester.

At your initial visit and again in month 9 when labor approaches, you will have an internal (pelvic) exam. You're probably familiar with these from your annual gynecological exams, but if you aren't, it's fairly straightforward. If the physician needs to visualize your cervix to perform a Pap smear, check for STDs, or check for amniotic fluid, a speculum (a duck-billed instrument) is inserted into your vagina and opened to form a tube through which your provider can view your vagina and cervix. It isn't painful, but you will probably experience some pressure that you may consider uncomfortable. He will also scrape off some cervical cells for a Pap smear and take a swab of vaginal fluid to test for sexually transmitted diseases. These also should not hurt.

Toward the very end of pregnancy, your doctor or midwife will again do an internal exam, this time to check the cervix for ripening—a sign of approaching labor.

Urine Tests

You'll be giving a urine sample for urinalysis at each prenatal visit. Your provider's office or lab will test your urine for ketones, protein, and glucose at each visit, and may also check for the presence of any bacteria. Depending on the protocol followed in your provider's office, you will be asked either to bring a fresh urine specimen to your appointment or provide one upon your arrival.

Ketones

Ketone bodies are substances produced when the body is getting insufficient fuel from food intake and has to metabolize fat for energy. The resulting ketosis process causes ketones to spill into the urine. Ketones may appear in pregnancy if you're suffering from severe nausea and vomiting, and they are signs that you may require intravenous nutrition. They can also be a byproduct of gestational diabetes when blood sugars are consistently high, and can lead to a rare but potentially life-threatening complication called *diabetic ketoacidosis* (DKA).

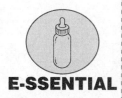

E-SSENTIAL

Your urine test is a good excuse to get some of those extra fluids your body and the baby need right now. Down a bottle of drinking water on the way to your checkup so that you can easily provide a sample, but don't overdo it or you may not make it without a pit stop.

The ketone test is generally performed with a reagent test strip, a strip of chemically treated paper that is dipped in your urine sample and then matched against a color chart for the presence of ketones. Test strips allow your provider or her staff to get almost instantaneous results.

If you have gestational diabetes, you will probably be prescribed a vial of ketone strips (Ketostix) for home use. Your provider will instruct you in their proper use.

Protein

Excessive protein (albumin) in the urine can be a sign of preeclampsia (also known as *toxemia*). It is also a possible indication of urinary tract infection (UTI) or of renal (kidney) impairment from chronic hypertension and/or diabetes. The presence of white blood cells in urine can be an indication of infection as well.

Your provider will again use a test strip to check for protein. If the strip is positive, it indicates that protein levels above 30 milligrams per deciliter (mg/dL) are detected; this is considered more than the trace amount normally present in urine. A positive protein strip is an indication for further testing with the more specific 24-hour urine test.

In a 24-hour urine test, you'll be given a special container in which to collect your urine, and you'll be asked to keep the sample refrigerated during the collection period (which ought to do wonders for your appetite). In a nonpregnant woman, 150 milligrams (mg) or less of total protein excreted in a day is considered normal; pregnant women typically excrete more, and a normal test in pregnancy is less than 300 mg for a 24-hour period.

If preeclampsia is suspected, your provider will probably order additional tests, including a blood draw, ultrasound, and fetal monitoring.

Glucose

Glucose (sugar) in the urine (called *glycosuria*) can be a sign of gestational diabetes mellitus (GDM). It's normal to spill a small amount of sugar into the urine in pregnancy, but consistently high levels along with other risk factors raise a red flag that GDM may be present. Again, test reagent strips (Diastix, Clinistix) are used for screening. If your doctor suspects gestational diabetes, he will order a 1-hour glucose challenge test.

Urine Culture

Your urine will be analyzed and cultured for the presence of bacteria at your first prenatal visit and again in the course of pregnancy if symptoms of a urinary tract infection appear (for example, burning during urination, strong-smelling urine). If you have certain conditions such as sickle cell anemia, a urine culture may be repeated throughout your pregnancy.

Blood Work

You won't be handing out your blood as frequently as your urine, but there are still a few blood tests involved in pregnancy.

Hemoglobin Count

Levels of hemoglobin, the red blood cells that carry oxygen throughout your body, will be assessed at your initial prenatal visit and may be tested again in the second and third trimesters. Low hemoglobin levels (called *anemia*) occur frequently in pregnancy due to the vast boost of your total blood volume. Levels that are too low can be a risk factor for low-birth-weight babies. If your total hemoglobin levels are below 12 mg/dL, your provider may prescribe iron supplements to build your hemoglobin reserves and may order regular hemoglobin screenings at each prenatal visit to monitor your progress.

Glucose Tests

Your doctor may give you a blood glucose test at your first prenatal visit to check for pre-existing type 2 diabetes, especially if you have risk factors for the condition. Risk factors include being overweight, being a member of a racial or ethnic group with a high prevalence of diabetes (that is, African American, Asian American, Hispanic, Native American, or Pacific Islander), having a history of previous gestational diabetes, a history of delivering a large baby, advanced maternal age, or a first-degree relative with diabetes. There are several variations of blood testing for diabetes, including a fasting plasma glucose test, a random plasma glucose test, and an A1C (hemoglobin A1C) test. If your results indicate diabetes, your provider will test you a second time to confirm.

E-ALERT!

High blood pressure (hypertension) results from an increase in the volume of fluid retained in the bloodstream, and the kidneys must work double time to clean and filter the blood. Eventually, skyrocketing blood pressure damages the nephrons (filtering units of the kidneys) and blood pressure rises further because the kidneys can't keep up.

Once you reach weeks 24 to 28 of pregnancy, your doctor will screen for gestational diabetes mellitus. ACOG endorses use of the glucose challenge test, which requires you to drink 50 grams of a glucose solution, a sugary flavored drink (usually Glucola). One hour later, blood will be drawn and your blood serum glucose levels will be measured. A level of 130 mg/dL or more is considered high. Some medical providers use a cutoff point of 140 mg/dL (ACOG endorses either). If your results exceed the cutoff levels, further testing with the oral glucose tolerance test (OGTT) will be necessary.

Oral Glucose Tolerance Test

Women with high serum glucose levels after the glucose challenge test must take an oral glucose tolerance test to establish a definitive diagnosis of gestational diabetes. The American Diabetes Association recommends use of the OGTT for all pregnant women in weeks 24 to 28 of pregnancy instead of the glucose challenge test.

The OGTT is a fasting test. You will be instructed not to eat for at least 8 hours prior to taking the test (usually midnight the evening before). Because pregnancy and fasting don't mix too well, especially if nausea is a problem for you, the test is typically administered first thing in the morning.

When you arrive at the lab, your blood will be drawn for a fasting reading. You will then be given 75 grams of Glucola to drink, and your blood will be taken again at the 1-hour and 2-hour marks. The glucose levels in the blood samples you provide will be analyzed and checked against the diagnostic criteria for GDM.

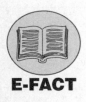

E-FACT

Some women find that their queasy stomachs simply can't tolerate Glucola—the sugary drink given for gestational diabetes screening. Two separate clinical studies published in the *American Journal of Obstetrics & Gynecology* have shown that jellybeans—a tastier alternative—are an effective stand-in for Glucola for women who experience side effects with the glucose solution.

The American Diabetes Association proposes the following criteria for a diagnosis of GDM.

Blood Sample	Criteria for GDM Diagnosis
Fasting	≥92 milligrams per deciliter, or mg/dL (5.1 millimoles per liter, or mmol/L)
1 hour	≥180 mg/dL (10 mmol/L)
2 hours	≥153 mg/dL (8.5 mmol/L)

NOTE: GDM is diagnosed when any one of these values is met or exceeded.

Other Blood Tests

Your blood type and Rhesus factor will be determined at your first prenatal visit. An Rh factor is either positive or negative. If your Rh is positive, no treatment is necessary. If you are Rh negative and your partner is Rh positive, you are at risk for Rh incompatibility with the blood type of your baby; this can occur when your unborn baby is Rh positive. If some of the baby's blood enters your bloodstream, your body may produce antibodies against the baby's blood, causing her to have severe anemia. When this happens, your immune system may try to fight off the baby as an intruder, causing serious complications. If caught early, however, the disorder can be treated effectively later in pregnancy.

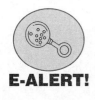

E-ALERT!

According to the March of Dimes, one in 2,000 women will develop chickenpox during pregnancy. This virus, known clinically as *varicella*, has the potential to cause birth defects if it is contracted during pregnancy. Fortunately, there are tests available to determine immunity to varicella; these may be given at the first prenatal appointment if you are unsure whether you have ever had the illness or the chicken pox vaccine.

Blood tests also determine whether you are immune to German measles (rubella). German measles can cause birth defects, especially if you contract the infection during the first trimester, and can cause cataracts, heart defects, and deafness in offspring. A majority of women have been exposed to the rubella virus or have been vaccinated against it before becoming pregnant. If you are not immune, you may be vaccinated following the delivery of the baby. Some women will not have immunity despite prior vaccination.

An HIV, hepatitis B, and syphilis test may also be done on your blood. Medications for HIV (human immunodeficiency virus) taken during pregnancy can decrease viral loads and practically eliminate transmission to the fetus in many cases. Treatment for syphilis can also prevent transmission to the fetus. If you test positive for hepatitis B, your baby will be vaccinated shortly after birth to protect him from the effects of hepatitis. He will receive the first three doses of the hepatitis B vaccine and hepatitis B immunoglobulin within 12 hours of birth to protect him from getting hepatitus B.

ACOG recommends that all pregnant couples be offered a blood test for cystic fibrosis screening.

Blood tests are also offered to screen for inherited sickle cell anemia in at-risk populations, including couples of African, Caribbean, Eastern Mediterranean, Middle Eastern, and Asian descent. Families of Greek, Italian, Turkish, African, West Indian, Arabian, or Asian descent may be screened for the thalassemia trait; if both father and mother are carriers, there is a chance that the fetus could develop the blood disease called *thalassemia major.*

The alpha-fetoprotein (AFP) test, usually part of a larger test called the *triple or quad screen*, is another blood test used in pregnancy to screen for genetic problems and certain birth defects. The AFP is described in more detail later in this chapter.

If initial blood-screening tests for genetic conditions are positive, further testing may help determine if a trait has been passed on to the baby. A trip to a genetic counselor to weigh all your options and assess their risks and benefits is a good idea.

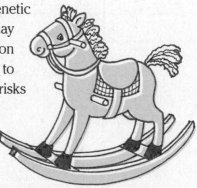

Swabs and Smears

More bodily fluid tests will be taken throughout pregnancy, particularly at the initial prenatal workup.

Pap Smear

Unless you've had one in the 12 months leading up to conception, your provider will take a Pap smear at your initial prenatal visit. During your pelvic exam, she will scrape a small sample of cells from your cervix using a spatula-like instrument. The cells are collected and sent to a lab for microscopic analysis.

An abnormal Pap smear result tells your doctor that something is going on with your cervix that requires further examination. Most abnormal Pap smears are caused by infection with a common, sexually transmitted virus known as the *human papilloma virus* (HPV). HPV may remain silent in women infected with the virus, causing no apparent symptoms. However, the virus can cause cellular changes on your cervix. While most of these changes will resolve on their own, some strains of HPV can cause cervical cancer if left untreated. Because of this, most women are regularly screened with Pap smears to detect any early changes that can be treated.

If your Pap smear is abnormal, you may be offered a colposcopy, a way of looking at your cervix with a microscope. Pregnancy should not prevent your colposcopy. However, an endocervical curettage (ECC), a scraping of the cervical canal routinely done as part of the colposcopy, should not be performed while you are pregnant.

Group B Strep

Group B streptococcus (GBS) is a bacterium that can cause serious infections in a newborn, including pneumonia and meningitis. If a pregnant woman tests positive for it, she is usually prescribed intravenous antibiotics during labor and delivery to prevent transmission to her baby.

Swabs of both the rectum and vagina are taken and cultured (put in a medium that will allow the bacteria to grow, if it is present). The Centers for Disease Control and Prevention (CDC) advise that all pregnant women be screened for GBS in weeks 35 to 37 of gestation.

Sexually Transmitted Infections (STIs)

The CDC also recommends that all pregnant women be screened for six sexually transmitted diseases—chlamydia, gonorrhea, hepatitis B, hepatitis C, HIV, and syphilis—because of their potentially devastating effects on a fetus. HIV, hepatitis B and C, and syphilis testing require a blood draw, while chlamydia and gonorrhea are tested by means of a vaginal swab sample followed by laboratory analysis. If you have a history of preterm delivery, your provider may also take a swab sample for bacterial vaginosis. You may only be offered some of these tests by your provider based on your medical history and perceived risk factors. If you'd like to be tested for all of them, ask your doctor.

Chlamydia, gonorrhea, and syphilis are caused by bacteria and can be treated with antibiotics. Viral infections like hepatitis B and HIV cannot be cured, but treatment and precautionary measures can greatly decrease the risk to your baby. HIV medications taken during pregnancy can lower viral loads and dramatically diminish the risk of transmission to the fetus, as can appropriate treatment for syphilis. If you test positive for hepatitis B, your baby will be vaccinated shortly after birth to protect him from the effects of hepatitis.

Ultrasounds

The test that most women look forward to—the ultrasound (sonogram)—gives you your first glimpse at your little one and lets your practitioner assess the baby's growth and development. It may also be used to diagnose placental abnormalities, an ectopic pregnancy, certain birth defects, or other suspected problems.

There are two types of ultrasound scans: the transabdominal, which scans through your abdomen, and the transvaginal, which scans through your vagina. In very early pregnancy, the technician may opt for the vaginal approach, which means that the transducer (handheld wand) will be inserted into your vagina. However, abdominal ultrasounds are the most common in that most ultrasounds take place in the second or third trimesters.

What to Expect

An ultrasound typically takes no longer than a half hour to perform. If you are in the first half of your pregnancy, you will probably be instructed to drink plenty of water prior to the exam and refrain from emptying your bladder. This is probably the most difficult part of the test. The extra fluids help the technician to visualize your baby.

Once in the examining room, you will recline on a table or bed with your upper body elevated and your abdomen exposed. Ask for extra pillows if you tend to get woozy when not lying on your side. The lights may be dimmed to allow the operator to see the sonogram picture more clearly. A thin application of transducer paste, jelly, or oil will be spread on your abdomen, and then the fun begins.

The ultrasound picture (sonogram) is obtained when high-frequency sound waves are passed over your abdomen with a transducer. These waves bounce off the solid structures of your baby, sending back a moving image of the tiny being inside. The resulting picture is transmitted to a computer or television screen.

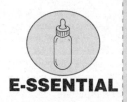

E-SSENTIAL

If your fetus isn't feeling coy on ultrasound day, a sonogram taken after 16 weeks may reveal its sex. A sighting of a little girl's labia (visible as three parallel lines) or a boy's penis can provide a fairly positive ID, but keep in mind that ultrasound is not foolproof and parents have been surprised in the delivery room.

The ultrasound technician may take a series of measurements during the procedure using the computer attached to the ultrasound unit. These measurements help your provider assess the growth and organ development of the fetus. Depending on the timing of the test and the cooperation of your unborn child, the provider may also be able to get an idea of the gender. Typically, this information won't be given unless you ask for it, in case you prefer to be surprised at birth.

Once the test is over, the technician will help you clean the transducer gel off your belly and you'll be able to empty your bladder if need be. The ultrasound operator can print out pictures for you to take home, so if she doesn't offer, make sure you ask.

A level-two ultrasound uses the same technology as a regular sonogram but involves a more detailed analysis of the results. It is frequently performed by a perinatologist who is specially trained in its use. The doctor will check fetal growth, organ system development, position of the placenta, and amniotic fluid volume. There are a number of reasons for a level-two to be ordered, from the routine to the potentially more serious. Your doctor should keep you informed, so if he hasn't given you a reason, ask.

Advances in Ultrasounds

Ultrasound pictures are typically a grainy black and white, but newer three-dimensional ultrasound technologies on the market can display your child in living (but simulated) color and are incredibly lifelike. The two-dimensional units are more common, however, in part because they are much less expensive.

The newest wave in ultrasound—four-dimensional technology—is actually 3D with movement added. The picture is clearer, and the movement component allows for diagnosis of heart defects. It can also be used to check for markers of developmentally normal fetal movements.

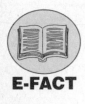

E-FACT

Although an estimated 70 percent of pregnant women in the United States currently have at least one ultrasound, ACOG does not currently support routine prenatal ultrasounds in low-risk pregnancies (except for specific medical indications). However, the routine use of ultrasounds is widespread outside of the United States.

When and if you have an ultrasound will depend upon your provider. Many obstetricians order ultrasounds as a matter of routine. Some do one at the first visit to check for correct dates and viability with the rationale that it may save them from questioning gestational dates later on (dating is more accurate when done in the first trimester). Others will recommend a sonogram at around week 20 to examine the fetal anatomy and ensure that the pregnancy is progressing normally.

A patient's peace of mind may also be reason enough to order an ultrasound. Since it is a noninvasive and fairly inexpensive test that can reassure the parents-to-be that matters are developing normally, many providers will comply with a woman's request for an ultrasound. If your doctor hasn't ordered one and you have some anxieties about your baby's health, it can't hurt to ask.

Alpha-fetoprotein (AFP)/Triple or Quad Screen Test

Alpha-fetoprotein is a protein produced by your unborn baby and passed into your circulatory system. The maternal serum AFP test, usually administered between weeks 15 and 18, is a blood test used to screen for chromosomal irregularities such as trisomy 18 and trisomy 21 (Down syndrome), and also for neural tube defects. It can also indicate the presence of twins, triplets, or more. Results of this test are usually available in about a week.

A more precise version of the AFP called the *triple screen test* (AFP-3) measures levels of hCG and estriol, a type of estrogen, as well as AFP. The quad test, an even more sensitive marker of chromosomal problems, assesses all three of these substances plus inhibin-A.

Most of the time, a high level of AFP is an indication of a multiples' gestation (twins, triplets, or more). However, it could also mean that your fetus has a neural tube defect. If AFP levels are low, it may be an indication of Down syndrome, trisomy 18, or other chromosomal disorders. A level-one or level-two ultrasound or an amniocentesis may be ordered for further evaluation. You may also be referred to a genetic counselor.

Keep in mind that a misdated pregnancy can also affect the results of your AFP or triple or quad screen and give a false positive. Ultrasound can help to confirm or adjust the gestational age.

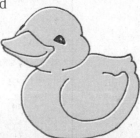

Amniocentesis

The thought of an amniocentesis makes many women nervous, probably because it involves two critical undertakings: a needle being inserted through the abdomen and breaching your baby's watery environment. It does carry some risk of complications, including a slight chance of miscarriage. However, the amnio (as it is commonly referred to) is one of the best tools available for diagnosing genetic disorders and chromosomal abnormalities. An amniocentesis is typically performed in the second trimester, sometime between weeks 15 and 20 of pregnancy. At this time, there are enough fetal cells present in the amniotic fluid for withdrawal and analysis. A later amnio may be done for various indications or reasons.

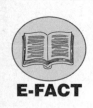

E-FACT

In addition to the wealth of genetic and health information it provides, an amnio can also tell you definitively if your baby is a boy or a girl. If you want to be surprised about the sex of your child, it may be a good idea to restate your wishes before you receive your amnio results.

Your provider may suggest that you meet with a genetic counselor prior to having an amniocentesis performed to weigh the risks versus the benefits of the procedure, given your specific medical background and family history. He will also lay out any alternative procedures that are options, such as a level-two ultrasound. If you do decide to go with the amnio, you might be sent to a perinatologist (maternal-fetal specialist) who is experienced in the procedure.

An amniocentesis is a relatively short outpatient procedure. First, an abdominal ultrasound is performed to look for an easily accessible pocket of amniotic fluid. Your abdomen is swabbed with an antiseptic solution, and the doctor will then insert a needle into the amniotic sac and draw an amniotic fluid sample into a syringe. The fluid contains sloughed-off fetal cells, which will be analyzed in the lab.

Here are reasons why an amniocentesis may be planned:

- **Age:** Women over age 35 have an increased risk of carrying a baby with a chromosomal disorder like Down syndrome. When the father is over 50, amniocentesis could also be advised because there may be a connection between paternal age and an increased risk of Down syndrome.
- **Family history:** If you've already had a baby with a hereditary or chromosomal abnormality or neural tube defects, or you or your partner have a family history of any of these conditions, an amniocentesis may be recommended.
- **Rh status:** Rh-negative women may have a amnio to determine the Rh status of their fetus. If your baby is Rh isoimmunized, trained professionals can administer an exchange blood transfusion through the fetal cord during an amniocentesis.
- **AFP, triple screen, or quad test results:** If your screen is abnormal, you may be offered an amnio.
- **Ultrasound abnormalities:** If your ultrasound turned up indications of the possibility of a chromosomal disorder, an amnio may be recommended for further evaluation.
- **Lung maturity:** If you're experiencing symptoms of preterm labor or other medical complications (placenta previa, prior classical C-section) that point to an early birth, your provider may perform an amnio to check for markers of fetal lung maturity.
- **Suspected intra-amniotic infection:** If you are experiencing preterm labor, you may be offered an amnio to rule out an intra-amniotic infection (a bacterial infection of the amniotic sac and the surrounding fluid).

After the amnio procedure, the baby will be monitored by ultrasound and will have his heart rate checked for a few minutes to ensure that everything is okay. Minimal cramping may follow the procedure. You will be advised to restrict strenuous exercise for a day (no step aerobics and no sex), although other normal activity should be fine. If in the days following amnio you experience fluid or blood discharge from the vagina, let your provider know as soon as possible.

The CDC estimates the chance of miscarriage following an amnio at somewhere between one in 400 and one in 200, and the risk of uterine infection at less than one in 1,000. There is also a slight risk of trauma to the unborn baby from a misplaced needle or inadvertent rupture of the sac.

If there are problems, the information you get from an amnio can prepare you for providing your child with the best possible care at birth. However, the timing can make other decisions difficult, such as whether to continue a pregnancy. Results from your amniocentesis won't be available for up to 2 weeks. And by the time the test results are back, you will be halfway through your pregnancy (about week 20). For this reason, some women at risk for chromosomal abnormalities will instead choose the chorionic villus sampling test, which can be performed in the first trimester.

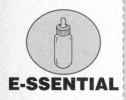

E-SSENTIAL

Some studies suggest that the experience and associated skill level of the physician performing a CVS or amniocentesis can make a big difference in the risk of complications. Many physicians will refer you to a specialist for just this reason. If your provider is performing the procedure, ask for an estimate of how many amnios or CVS procedures she has performed.

Chorionic Villus Sampling (CVS)

CVS stands for *chorionic villus sampling*, a test performed in the first trimester (usually in weeks 10 to 12) to assess chromosomal abnormalities and hereditary conditions in the unborn baby. Your provider will use ultrasound guidance to insert a catheter into the placenta, either through the cervix (transcervical) or through a needle injected into the abdomen (transabdominal). The catheter is used to extract a biopsy (sample) of the tiny chorionic villi, the fingers of tissue surrounding the embryo that are the beginnings of the placenta. The villi are a genetic match for the baby's own tissue.

Slight cramping and spotting are normal after the procedure, and you will probably be advised to indulge in some rest and relaxation for the remainder of the day. If bleeding continues, is excessive, or is accompanied by pain or fever, call your practitioner immediately.

E-ALERT!

A CVS is not always accurate. The exact spot where the technician removes the cell sampling from the chorion can be critical. Also, some abnormalities in chorionic tissues do not always show up in the fetus. Ask for clarification or a second opinion of any negative (that is to say, normal) CVS report before you decide on any course of action in your pregnancy.

CVS has several benefits over amnio. It can be performed earlier (first trimester as opposed to second), and the results are available much faster (5 to 7 days for preliminary CVS results versus 10 to 14 days for amnio). However, the risk of miscarriage is higher with CVS—between one in 200 and one in 100 will experience miscarriage after the procedure. The risk is higher for women with a retroverted (tipped or tilted) uterus who are given a transcervical CVS (about five in 100). For this reason, a transabdominal CVS (through the abdominal wall) is usually advised for these women. A consultation with a genetic counselor can help you analyze the positives and negatives and decide whether a CVS is right for you.

Fetal Monitoring

A fetal heart monitor measures—you guessed it—the fetal heart rate (FHR). A baseline (average) fetal heart rate of 120 to 160 beats per minute (bpm) is considered normal. During your routine prenatal exams, a handheld monitor is used to quickly listen to the fetal heart rate. If you need to be monitored for a longer period of time, belts are used to keep the monitors in place for a period of about 20 minutes. Your health care provider will look for fetal heart rate accelerations, which correspond to your baby's movement and are a sign of fetal well-being. Reasons to have the prolonged monitoring include going past your due date, intrauterine growth restriction (IUGR), gestational diabetes, and other medical conditions.

During Labor

There is some controversy over the need to monitor the baby's heart rate during labor. Some health care providers prefer to measure the heart rate continuously, while others will use the monitor intermittently. For high-risk pregnancies and inductions of labor, continuous fetal monitoring is generally preferred.

There are both external and internal uterine monitors available. An external monitor provides information on the frequency and length of contractions, while an internal monitor provides this as well as information on the contractions' strength.

External monitors are held in place using two belts around your belly. The transducers on each are adjusted until they are both measuring your contractions and picking up the fetal heart sounds. If you are in a high-risk pregnancy, you may be hooked up to an internal fetal monitor during labor and delivery. Internal monitors are only used in labor when the amniotic sac has broken. This monitor is considered more sensitive and accurate but is also more constricting. It uses a little springlike wire that is inserted

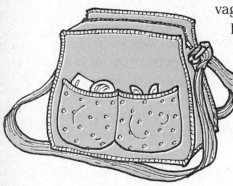

vaginally and is placed just under the skin on the baby's head. The wires are secured to the mother's leg using tape or special sticky pads.

Both internal and external monitoring can keep you tethered to your bed during labor, which may not be the experience you want. External monitors can be removed for a short time, but in general fetal movement should be assessed at least every 15 minutes. A newer type of monitor that uses telemetry allows some women to go wireless during labor.

Stress and Nonstress Tests (NST)

If there is any concern about fetal well-being or if you are still waiting for baby's belated arrival at week 41 or 42, you'll probably be given a nonstress test (NST) to measure fetal heart rate. It is performed any time after week 26.

The NST is administered while you are lying on a bed or examining table and are attached to a fetal monitor. The monitor belts are strapped around your abdomen. For about 20 minutes, every time you feel your baby move, you'll push a button. The button will record the baby's heartbeat on the paper strip or computer record. Depending on how the monitor is hooked up, the monitor may also detect and note the baby's movement. Rises in the FHR should correspond to fetal movement.

If there is no movement, it's quite possible that baby is sleeping; you'll be given a drink of juice or a small snack in an attempt to rouse her. Sometimes a buzzer or vibrations called *vibroacoustic stimulation* (VAS) are used to wake up a sleeping fetus. If these methods are unsuccessful, further tests including an ultrasound may be ordered.

In a stress test (also called a *contraction stress test* or *oxytocin challenge test*), mild contractions are induced with the synthetic hormone Pitocin to see how your baby responds. You will be hooked up to a fetal monitor, and you will receive an injection of Pitocin (synthetic form of the oxytocin hormone). If the baby cannot maintain his heartbeat during a contraction, immediate delivery may be indicated (possibly by C-section).

Biophysical Profile (BPP)

A biophysical profile (BPP) is simply an ultrasound combined with a non-stress test. A BPP assesses fetal heart rate, muscle tone, body and breathing movement, and the amount of amniotic fluid. The test takes about a half hour. A low BPP score may indicate that the fetus is getting insufficient oxygen. If the fetal lungs are mature, immediate delivery may be recommended.

Women in high-risk pregnancies may undergo regular weekly or biweekly BPP testing in the third trimester. BPP is also a standard test for a post-term pregnancy—one that has gone beyond 42 weeks. Your physician may also order a modified biophysical profile, which is a BPP that consists of the NST and an ultrasound assessment of amniotic fluid only (the amniotic fluid index, AFI).

Genetic Counseling

If you have a history of genetic disease or birth defects in your family or are considered at risk for passing along a hereditary disorder based on your ethnic or racial background, your provider may refer you for genetic counseling, another tool in the prenatal diagnostic arsenal. Genetic counselors certified by the American Board of Genetic Counseling have a "CGC" designation after their names, which indicates that they have passed a certification exam, have a graduate degree in genetic counseling, and have logged significant clinical training experience.

What It Is

A genetic counselor takes a detailed family and social history and creates a statistical analysis of your child's risk for acquiring genetic or birth defects. She will also provide you with information on the conditions in question and the risks and benefits of further testing and will answer any questions you may have. Some of these tests may involve checking you or your partner for carrier genes, while others test the fetus.

What It Isn't

Some women refuse genetic counseling on the grounds that they would never elect to terminate their pregnancy. However, genetic counseling isn't designed to be a survival-of-the-fittest venture but rather a way to help you and your partner reach an informed decision. A genetic counselor is trained to remain objective and not to attempt to influence your choices. Many couples can and do continue a pregnancy even after testing indicates their child will be born with a serious medical condition or birth defect. Advance knowledge allows a family to prepare emotionally and to create a suitable environment for a special-needs newborn. It can also mean a better outcome for the child to have a medical support network already in place.

Chronic Health Conditions

If you have a chronic health problem such as diabetes, asthma, or heart disease, you will face some special challenges over the next 9 months as your body adjusts to the major remodeling going on internally. Remember that your baby's health depends on your well-being, so staying on top of your treatment is essential. It's important to bring your primary health care provider into the pregnancy picture as soon as possible (ideally, when you start planning your pregnancy).

Your doctor may adjust your medication or treatment regimen and in most cases will want to follow your progress closely. You may also be referred to a perinatologist—an ob-gyn who specializes in high-risk pregnancies. Your primary care provider and any specialists should remain an integral part of your health care team throughout your pregnancy. Any changes to your treatment should be made in consultation with your doctors, and likewise your perinatologist should be notified of any significant changes they make in your treatment during your pregnancy. Open communication during this critical time is absolutely essential; if any of your providers isn't willing to be a team player, find someone who is.

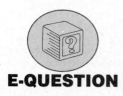

E-QUESTION

I'm forty. What are my chances of an uncomplicated pregnancy?
Women over age 35 have a higher risk for developing diabetes, high blood pressure, and placental problems in pregnancy. There is also an increased risk of having a baby with a chromosomal disorder. The good news is that proper prenatal care can greatly reduce your risk of these complications.

You will be making more frequent visits to all of your health care providers throughout pregnancy to ensure that your illness remains well controlled and is not adversely affecting your unborn child. Any conditions that may potentially be transmitted to your child (for example, HIV, herpes) either in the womb or during delivery may require drug therapy and/or potential cesarean section.

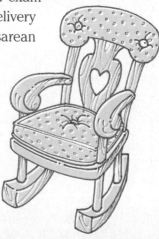

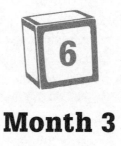

Month 3

This is a landmark month as you finish up your first trimester. You start to sport a bump, which makes your pregnancy visible to the outside world. If you haven't shared your news with friends, family, and coworkers, now is the time—before they start asking questions. Your little fetus is growing by leaps and bounds, and you make first contact this month as you hear her heartbeat and perhaps even see her on ultrasound.

Baby This Month

By the end of this month, baby will grow to over 2 inches in length and almost 1 ounce, about the size and heft of a roll of Life Savers. If you could look at his face, you'd see that his ears and closed eyelids have now fully developed. His head accounts for one-third of his total length, and his tongue, salivary glands, and taste buds have also formed. Even though he's a long way from his first meal, studies indicate he may already be getting a taste of what you've been snacking on from the amniotic fluid.

He is now getting all of his nutrients through the fully formed placenta (from the Greek *plakuos*, meaning *flat cake*, its approximate shape), an organ that you and your fetus share. The umbilical cord tethers the fetus to the placenta, which provides it with nutrients and oxygen and transports waste materials away.

E-FACT

As you enter the second trimester, your risk of miscarriage drops dramatically. While an estimated 15 percent of recognized pregnancies result in miscarriage in the first trimester, by the time you hear your baby's heartbeat around week 12, the risk of miscarriage for most women drops to 1 to 5 percent.

Your baby's heart is pumping about 25 quarts of blood each day, and a lattice of blood vessels can be seen through her translucent skin, which is starting to develop a coat of fine downy hair called *lanugo*. The gender is apparent because the external sex organs have now fully differentiated, but it will take a combination of luck and technical skill for an ultrasound technician to reveal whether you have a son or daughter.

Your Body This Month

You probably never thought you'd be pleased by a potbellied profile, but this significant, visible sign of your pregnancy is a landmark moment for many women. Wear it proudly. You've taken your child through the first 3 critical months of growth, and your belly is a badge of honor that tells the world about this important accomplishment.

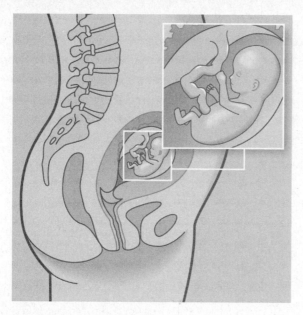

You and your fetus
at the end of the first
trimester

Your Body Changes

Your uterus is about the size of a softball and stretches to just about your pubic bone. Four to six pounds of total weight gain is about average for the first trimester; if you've been down and out with nausea and vomiting, you may be below the curve. Weight gain will pick up in the second trimester and peak in the third as your baby starts to fill out your womb.

Don't take the "eating for two" cliché literally: 300 extra calories per day is about all you'll require to meet your baby's nutritional needs. Gaining too much can exacerbate the aches and pains of pregnancy, place an extra strain on your back, increase the risk of having a large baby, and put you at risk for hypertension (high blood pressure) and gestational diabetes. On the other hand, if you find the aversions and nausea of pregnancy have you keeping down only a certain type of not-so-nutritious food (pepperoni pizza, for example), don't feel bad about it. The most important thing right now is keeping some food down and your energy up. Try experimenting with healthier variations if your stomach will take it (skip the pepperoni in exchange for extra cheese or veggies), and hang in there. By the end of the first trimester, most women report that their morning sickness gets better or (fingers crossed) completely disappears.

E-ALERT!

What You Feel Like

Although nausea and vomiting may finally be waning thanks to a decline in hCG levels, you may find that constipation, gas, and occasional heartburn take over as the gastrointestinal pests of the second trimester. Constipation is caused by an increase in progesterone, which can slow down the digestive system. Later in the pregnancy, pressure on the intestine caused by your growing uterus adds to the problem.

Iron supplements or prenatal vitamins with added iron can also cause constipation, so talking to your provider about the possibility of a dosage adjustment or an extended release formula may be in order. An increase in dietary fiber, plenty of water intake, and exercise as approved by your health care provider may also help to get your system going again. Be sure to consult your doctor before taking any stool softeners or laxatives.

Gas may become a source of discomfort and occasional embarrassment as well. Consider cutting back on foods that worsen the problem (for example, onions, beans, broccoli, cabbage, carbonated drinks). Fiber you take to eliminate constipation can also aggravate gas problems. To keep the burps at bay, try small, frequent snacks instead of large meals.

Other pregnancy symptoms that may continue or begin this month include:

- ✓ Fatigue
- ✓ Frequent urination
- ✓ Tender breasts
- ✓ Occasional dizziness or faintness
- ✓ Headaches

At Your Doctor Visit

Make sure your husband or partner makes this month's prenatal appointment. You're both in for a treat as you begin to experience the sights and sounds of your growing child.

Tests This Month

Depending on your provider's policy on ultrasound exams and on your personal medical history, you may be seeing your baby this month.

Your provider will also start estimating the size of your baby by taking a tape measure to your belly and counting the centimeters from your pubic bone to the tip of your fundus—the top of your uterus. Taking this measurement at each visit gives your practitioner a way to assess your baby's ongoing growth. Some practitioners do not take the fundal height until after week 12 or even week 20. It's important to remember that fundal height is used as a screening tool only; women who are overweight, carrying multiples, or have a fetus in the breech position may not measure accurately.

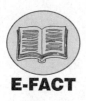

E-FACT

If the fundal height is too large or too small for gestational age, it could indicate problems such as gestational diabetes or intrauterine growth retardation. After 20 weeks of pregnancy, the length in centimeters should be roughly equivalent to the baby's gestational age in weeks, give or take 3 centimeters.

You may be told about the alpha-fetoprotein test or triple/quad screen this month. This blood test is typically given in weeks 15 to 18 and screens for the possibility of neural tube defects and/or chromosomal abnormalities in the fetus. Since the test is optional, many providers give an informational sheet to patients the month before so that they have time to consider whether they want to take it.

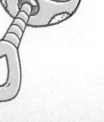

Baby's Heartbeat

Hearing the steady woosh-woosh of your baby's heart for the first time is one of the most thrilling and emotional moments of pregnancy. Your first chance happens this month as your provider checks for the fetal heartbeat, using a small ultrasound device called a Doppler or Doptone. If you have a retroverted uterus (tipped or tilted), it's possible the Doppler won't detect the heartbeat just yet. Don't be alarmed; by your next prenatal appointment you will probably be able to hear it loud and clear.

On Your Mind

This month you are dealing with an expanding belly and new body shape, and you may also be dealing with forgetfulness.

Forgetfulness

Have you walked around looking for your sunglasses for 20 minutes before finding them on your head? Lost your car keys for the fifth time this week? Like any mom-to-be, you've got a lot on your mind. That alone may have you forgetting details that used to be second nature and misplacing items. Although researchers have looked at the problem of memory impairment in pregnancy, there hasn't been a clear consensus on the definitive cause. Pregnancy hormones, sleep deprivation, and stress have all been suggested as possible culprits.

Some studies have suggested that impairments in working memory, the short-term spatial memory you use to remember things like where you parked at the grocery store, are related to excessive levels of estrogen that start in pregnancy and peak in the third trimester. In other words, your forgetfulness might be hanging around a few more months. Until then, think about carrying a small notebook with you as a memory crutch. This can keep you from losing your mind—and your car.

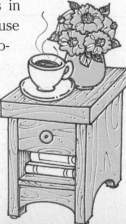

Whatever the cause, forgetting appointments and misplacing things can leave you feeling muddled and helpless. Try relying less on your memory by writing notes, sticking to a routine (for example, car keys always go into a basket by the door), and living by a written or electronic organizer. If you aren't the wired type, start requesting a 24-hour advance phone call reminder when you schedule service appointments such as in-home appliance repair or a salon appointment. Having a system—whatever it is—is the key to staying reasonably organized and mentally together during this hectic time.

Feeling Good about Your Changing Body

A word on weight: try not to get too hung up on it. Stepping on the scale at every doctor visit can make body weight seem like a pass-or-fail test, but this is just one tool your provider has to make sure your baby is growing on schedule. Don't dread the regular weigh in; look on it as tangible proof that your unborn child is growing and developing well.

E-ALERT!

Never diet in pregnancy, even if you've already gained more than expected. Restricting calorie and nutrient intake can hamper fetal development. If you're concerned about excessive weight gain, consider seeing a registered dietitian for help with meal planning and/or taking a provider-approved prenatal exercise class.

Further, don't compare your pregnancy body weight to those who have gone before you. If older neighbors, friends, and relatives remark on their own minimal weight gain and quick return to prepregnancy weight, there's a reason. Up through the 1970s, ideal pregnancy weight gains averaged 10 to 15 pounds less than they do today, according to the Institute of Medicine. Studies have since shown that weight gain should be individualized to a mother's prepregnancy body mass index (BMI) and that inadequate weight gain can contribute to low-birth-weight babies.

Now is a good time to go out and buy that first maternity outfit if you haven't already done so. Pick out something comfortable and stylish that makes you feel good—and maybe even shows off your belly a bit.

Spreading the Word

Now that you're showing, keeping your pregnancy to yourself is difficult. If you and your partner have kept the good news to yourselves so far—for a whole trimester, no less—this is probably the time to spill it.

Sharing with Friends and Family

How you tell your parents, siblings, and best friends that you and your partner are pregnant can be one of the most exciting moments of pregnancy. It can also be a little nerve-racking if you're not sure how the news will be received.

If you've held off sharing your pregnancy until now, "Why did you wait so long to tell us?" might be a common refrain. Whatever your reasons for waiting have been, they're valid. Let your family and friends know they're important to you, which is why you've chosen to make them the first outside of your partner to know about your new addition. (See Chapter 11 for hints about informing your kids.)

Some fun ideas for sharing the news with parents, friends, and others:

- Give them an ultrasound picture (or a photocopy of one), and let it explain itself.
- Send out birthday invitations for the estimated due date.
- Take out a "Help Wanted: Grandparents" advertisement in their local classifieds and point the prospective grandparents to it.
- Invite them to dinner (at home or out) and serve a frosting-inscribed "It's a Boy/Girl/Fetus," "Congratulations, Auntie," or "We're Pregnant" cake for dessert.
- Ask your mom or sister to go shopping with you, and take her to your 3-month ob-gyn appointment instead.
- If this isn't your first child, let your kids spread the news in their own special ways.
- The old standby "Guess what?" works well, too.

Alas, there are some people in the world who are perpetually in a glass-half-empty state of mind. Perhaps you are related to one. If you expect a negative reaction from someone who must be clued in to the pregnancy (read: immediate family member), try to take along your spouse or partner for emotional support. You can hope that the proverbial wet blanket will surprise you both with a hug and well-wishes. If not, treat yourself to a date with your partner and let it go as a character defect.

When (and What) to Tell Your Workplace

Now that your pregnancy is visible and your doctor's appointments are taking you away from your workplace on a regular basis, it is a good time to let your employer in on your secret. From a practical viewpoint, you'll want to find out about your company's leave policy, maternity benefits, and health insurance coverage for new family members.

So, how do you break the news? Make sure you tell your supervisor or manager first. Hearing about your impending maternity leave through the grapevine could make your manager question your commitment to your career. Go into the meeting with an idea of how much maternity leave you'd like to take and, even better, of who might cover your job responsibilities while you're away.

If you're asked about your plans after baby is born, be honest while playing your cards close to your chest. If you're happy with your career and workplace but unsure whether your tune will change once you see your darling son or daughter, let your employer know you have every intention of returning to work and leave it at that. Disingenuous? Not at all. You can't give a definitive response to a situation that hasn't even occurred yet. That's like asking your employer to make a hiring decision on an applicant he hasn't interviewed yet. You can, however, give him your assurances that you're pleased with your position, if that's the case.

On the other hand, if you've already decided that motherhood will be your new full-time vocation, quitting right after your maternity leave runs out with no fair warning to your supervisor is a sure-fire way to burn bridges and ruin a reference. Check out whether you can be switched over to your spouse's health insurance now, and take other appropriate steps to give your employer ample notice to find a replacement. If you're worried about losing your job

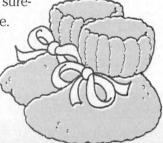

before you're ready to leave, let your supervisor know how long you'd like to work and point out the advantages of your using the time remaining to train your replacement.

Just for Dads

A boy to bond with or a girl to graduate magna cum laude from Harvard? You and your significant other have now been thinking about the prospect of a son or daughter, especially if you have an ultrasound appointment approaching. If you're going to try to find out the gender of your child, keep an open mind since you have little choice in the matter. Think instead of the exceptional beauties and joys to be found in both sexes as well as any special sibling relationships that can be forged. More important, start thinking of your baby in terms of human potential rather than through gender-imposed limitations; after all, girls can carry on the family name just as readily as boys.

Speaking of names, you have probably already started to think about names for the little one. Below are the most popular names for babies born in 2010.

▼ THE TEN MOST POPULAR U.S. BABY NAMES FOR 2010

Boys' Names	Girls' Names
Jacob	Isabella
Ethan	Sophia
Michael	Emma
Jayden	Olivia
William	Ava
Alexander	Emily
Noah	Abigail
Daniel	Madison
Aiden	Chloe
Anthony	Mia

Source: U.S. Social Security Administration

The Cost of Kids

Worried about how to make ends meet as your family grows? Sit down with your significant other and work through a budget together. Chances are there's room for cutting back on entertainment and those weekend getaways that you won't be taking for a while anyway after the baby is born.

Still concerned that you won't bring home enough income to support your family? Consider the pregnancy as a new beginning for yourself as well. If you've been thinking about making a career move, spiff up your resume and network now, while your household is still relatively quiet. Even if you really love your present job, finding out what else is out there and getting an offer on the table can give you leverage in negotiating with your current employer.

Changing Roles

You, a dad? The same guy whose idea of a savings account is 6 months' worth of bar change filling a water cooler bottle? The guy who still collects *Star Wars* action figures (ahem, collectibles)? Who still calls his dad when the car acts up and has 20 more years of student loan payments ahead of him? It's hard to grasp until you experience it, but the sense of responsibility, intense love, and fierce protectiveness that are part of parenthood will make you feel more of an adult than probably any event in your life thus far. Believe it or not, some day that little boy or girl will be calling you for automotive advice (and playing with your collectibles).

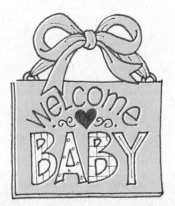

Eating Right

If you're like more than three-quarters of American women, you probably weren't eating enough fruits and vegetables before your pregnancy. And odds are that you also weren't getting enough magnesium and vitamins E, A, and C. Pregnancy provides the perfect opportunity to evaluate and reinvent your dietary habits. Unfortunately, morning sickness, heartburn, and other pregnancy discomforts can sabotage your best intentions. Don't be discouraged. Open your mind and palate to new nutrient-rich foods, and be flexible with the size and frequency of your meals.

Healthy Diet, Healthy Womb, Healthy Baby

Recent research into fetal development has established that a mother's diet at conception and throughout pregnancy has a direct impact on her child's health in infancy and beyond. Babies who are undernourished in pregnancy are at risk for low birth weight, and low-birth-weight infants have an increased risk of chronic disease later in life—specifically heart disease, hypertension, stroke, and type 2 diabetes.

Throughout pregnancy, your baby will be receiving nutrients from two primary sources—the food you eat and the nutrient stores in your body. The placenta is the pipeline for baby's growth, funneling nutrients to the fetus and taking waste products out. Depending on your nutritional state before and during pregnancy, and the gender of your baby (boys tend to grow faster), your placenta may expand in surface area to compensate for any missing nutrients in your diet.

Your best strategy for a healthy baby and body is to eat a well-balanced, nutrient-dense diet with sufficient caloric intake. You should also take prenatal supplements. Even if you're experiencing morning sickness, the supplements should help compensate for any nutritional shortcomings.

Prenatal Nutrition Basics

In pregnancy, women require an extra 300–350 calories above their normal daily intake to meet the needs of their growing babies. The quality of those calories is particularly important; your developing child requires an extra boost of a variety of vitamins and minerals. Most of these nutrients are best served through your regular diet. Start making it a habit to check nutrition labels in the grocery store and invest in a good pocket-sized nutrition guide to help you choose produce and other unlabeled items. However, you will probably require a supplement to meet your iron needs, which nearly double in pregnancy (to 27 mg daily).

It's important to eat a well-balanced diet rich in nutrients. This is usually best achieved by eating a variety of "whole," or unprocessed, foods. The USDA and ACOG suggest the following general dietary guidelines for each food group.

▼ RECOMMENDED DAILY FOOD CHOICES IN PREGNANCY

Food Group	Daily Servings	Tips for Smart Choices
Bread, Cereal, Rice, and Pasta Group	6 ounces	Choose whole grains
Fruit Group	2 cups	Fresh fruits are best
Meat, Poultry, Fish, Dry Beans, Eggs, and Nuts Group	5.5 ounces	Select lean cuts. Vary your choices
Milk, Yogurt, and Cheese Group	3 cups	Choose low-fat and fat-free. If you are lactose intolerant, take a calcium supplement
Vegetable Group	2.5 cups	Have a mix of orange and dark green veggies and dried beans and peas
Oils and Solid Fats	Use sparingly	Healthy fats come from fish, nuts, and vegetable oils

Based on a 2,000 calorie diet. Talk to your health care provider about the dietary plan that's right for you and your baby.

Vitamins and Supplements

Iron helps to manufacture an adequate supply of hemoglobin—important for pregnant moms, who experience a 40 to 50 percent increase in blood volume during pregnancy. Your unborn baby is also storing iron that will last for the first few months of life outside your womb. Baby takes what she needs from your store of iron first, so she won't suffer if your intake is inadequate. However, you will end up with anemia, a red-blood-cell deficiency that can make you feel tired and makes it harder for your blood to carry oxygen throughout your body and to the baby. To combat anemia, eat a variety of iron-rich foods like liver, red meat, fish, poultry, enriched breads and cereals, leafy green vegetables, eggs, and dried fruits. Your health care provider will recommend an iron-enriched prenatal vitamin or iron supplement to make up for any deficiency.

Take iron supplements between meals with plenty of water to eliminate some of the common side effects, like constipation, diarrhea, and nausea. Although taking iron supplements between meals promotes better absorption, if you're suffering from morning sickness and find it difficult to keep your supplements down, you should try taking them with a meal. If constipation is a problem, add prune juice or other high-fiber sources to your diet.

To enhance absorption of iron, take your supplement with a fruit juice rich in ascorbic acid (vitamin C), such as orange juice. Remember that tea and coffee contain substances that can inhibit your absorption of iron (as well as calcium), so try to avoid using these to wash down supplements or as an accompaniment to iron-rich foods.

Another critical nutrient in pregnancy is folic acid (folate), which significantly lowers your baby's risk of developing neural tube defects (birth defects of the brain and spinal cord, such as spinal bifida and anencephaly). Because the neural tube forms during the first 4 weeks of pregnancy—before many women even realize they are pregnant—the CDC recommends that all women of childbearing age get at least 400 micrograms (mcg) of folic acid daily. Pregnant women and women planning a pregnancy should get more: 600 mcg daily of folic acid in food or supplement form.

Foods rich in folate include orange juice, enriched breads and grain products, leafy green vegetables, and dried beans. Since 1998 the FDA has required that grain products such as enriched breads, pastas, rice, and cornmeal also be fortified with this important nutrient. Today there are dozens of breakfast cereals on the market that contain 100 percent of the daily value of folic acid, and just one bowl each morning can make a big difference in your baby's health. Most prenatal vitamins also include the recommended daily allowance (RDA) of folic acid.

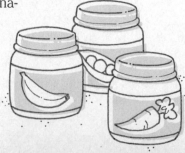

▼ **WOMEN'S RECOMMENDED DAILY ALLOWANCES IN PREGNANCY**

Calories	+300
Calcium	1,000 mg (milligrams)
Folate	600 mcg (micrograms)
Iron	27 mg
Magnesium	350–360 mg
Niacin	18 mg
Riboflavin	1.4 mg
Selenium	60 mcg
Thiamin	1.4 mg
Vitamin A	770 mcg
Vitamin B_6	1.9 mg
Vitamin B_{12}	2.6 mcg
Vitamin C	85 mg
Vitamin E	15 mg
Vitamin K	90 mcg
Zinc	11 mg

Recommended daily intake from food and supplement sources combined.

Source: Food and Nutrition Board, Institute of Medicine, National Academy of Sciences; Dietary Reference Intake Tables.

If you aren't a numbers person or if you feel overwhelmed by the thought of logging every item that passes your lips, don't worry. Take your prenatal supplement as prescribed by your doctor to bank those vitamins and minerals, then follow a few simple guidelines to ensure that you and baby get your daily fuel.

Confused by all the "guidelines" and just want someone to tell you what to eat? Visit the USDA's online menu planner at *www.choosemyplate.gov* and customize a food plan for pregnancy. Keep copies on your refrigerator, in your bag, or anywhere else that will be easily accessible when you make meal choices. Then use the serving suggestions as a minimum guide for a balanced, healthy diet. Be sure to touch base with your provider about how your individual nutrition needs vary if you have a food allergy or other health condition requiring a special diet.

Weight Gain—The Facts

Although 25 to 35 pounds is the average total weight gain suggested for a pregnancy, your height and build will influence that number. Underweight women and women carrying multiples are expected to gain more (28 to 40 pounds); overweight women are encouraged to gain slightly less (15 to 25 pounds). If your provider hasn't mentioned a weight goal for your pregnancy, ask him what his expectations are.

On average, women only gain about 2 to 4 pounds in the first trimester (sometimes less if morning sickness has been a problem). Weight gain typically picks up in the second trimester and peaks in the third. See the table that follows for a breakdown of where pregnancy weight is distributed in your body.

It's important to avoid letting the scale become an obsession. Focus instead on the quality of food you're eating and on getting some regular exercise (cleared with your provider first). Your health and your baby's health are the goals of this pregnancy.

▼ **BREAKDOWN OF WHERE THE WEIGHT GOES**

Baby	7.5 to 8.5 pounds
Uterus	2 to 2.5 pounds
Placenta	1.5 to 2 pounds
Amniotic fluid	2 pounds
Blood	3 to 4 pounds
Breasts	1 to 2 pounds
Maternal fat and nutrient stores	4 to 6 pounds
Retained maternal fluids	4 to 8 pounds

Eating Through Morning Sickness

If you're dealing with morning sickness, eating healthfully (and keeping it down) is a particular challenge. Your stomach will have definite opinions on what it will and will not tolerate; when you're feeling nauseated, let it guide you. Stick to what works—even if it's the same thing three times daily. Morning sickness won't last forever, and prenatal vitamins will help even-out your nutrient intake while you get through this difficult period. Don't worry if you don't gain weight in the first trimester due to morning sickness. It's more important to have weight gain in the following trimester.

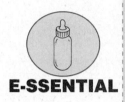

You may find yourself snacking more in pregnancy, either to keep morning sickness at bay or because your growing baby is leaving less room for a full stomach. Mini-meals can also help combat indigestion and heartburn. Try snacks that pack a protein punch such as peanut butter on whole-wheat crackers or yogurt with wheat germ swirled in.

Preparing meals when you're not feeling well can be even more challenging than eating them, so try to get help in the kitchen from your spouse or significant other, if possible. If not, stock up on foods that require minimal prep work, such as frozen entrees and canned soups, so that you can eat with little effort.

As you have likely already discovered, both the taste and the smell of fatty and spicy foods can aggravate an already sensitive stomach, so try to stick to some bland basics. Traditional comfort foods nourish many women suffering through morning sickness; staples like soup, rice, pasta, and potatoes can be a filling way to get needed calories.

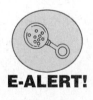

Strong odors can be a morning-sickness trigger for many women. You may want to avoid cooking foods right now that pack a fragrant punch, like fish, onions, and cabbage. If you can't avoid doing so, turn on the kitchen exhaust fan and open a window. Cooking strong-smelling foods in the microwave also helps to minimize the odor.

Changing your meal patterns to small but more frequent snacks can make eating more tolerable. Remember that low blood sugar is a nausea trigger, so the worst thing you can do for your morning sickness is to skip meals. And you need those calories and nutrients for that growing baby!

Dehydration can also contribute to nausea. If drinking fluids makes your stomach turn, opt for foods with a high fluid content, such as frozen juice bars, grapes, and melon.

Foods to Avoid

As a rule of thumb, now that you're "eating for two" all meat prepared to order should be well-done, and shellfish, fish, fowl, and eggs should be thoroughly cooked to avoid parasites and pathogens. Some food-borne pathogens are easier to acquire while pregnant, and food-borne illnesses have the potential to cause vomiting, nausea, and dehydration that could put your baby at risk. Some foods should be completely off the menu during pregnancy. These include:

✓ **Anything with raw eggs as an ingredient.** Some items you may not think of as hazardous are off limits, such as uncooked cake batter and cookie dough, hollandaise sauce and Caesar salad dressing (check the labels or ask your waiter about the eggs), eggnog, and even undercooked scrambled eggs (unless prepared with pasteurized eggs, as is commercial cookie dough ice cream).

✓ **Deli luncheon meats and hot dogs.** Luncheon meats—both those from the deli and those that are prepackaged—can harbor the harmful bacteria *listeria*. Raw hot dogs can also contain strains of listeria. You *can* eat these meats if you heat them to steaming (at least 165°F), which will kill the bacteria.

✓ **King mackerel, swordfish, shark, and tilefish.** All four can contain high levels of mercury that is potentially harmful to a baby's developing brain. Additionally, the FDA suggests limiting all fish to two servings (12 ounces) per week during pregnancy and while breastfeeding.

✓ **Refrigerated pâtés, meat spreads, and smoked seafood.** Pâtés that require refrigeration can harbor the *listeria* bacteria.

✓ **Some soft cheeses.** Brie, Camembert, feta, Mexican-style, and blue-veined soft cheeses can also carry the *listeria* bacteria. The FDA does not allow the importation or sale of unpasteurized cheese unless aged for 60 days or more. However, use caution if traveling out of the country.

✓ **Sprouts.** Steer clear of raw vegetable sprouts (for example, alfalfa, radish), which may carry *E. coli* bacteria.

✓ **Sushi.** Again, uncooked fish can be hazardous to your health. Substitute California rolls.

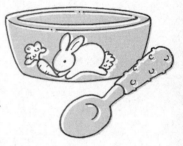

✓ **Unpasteurized juice or dairy.** Any dairy or juice product not clearly marked as "pasteurized" should be avoided.

Kitchen Safety

Proper storage and handling of food, from the supermarket to your dinner table, is the best way to combat food-borne illness in your kitchen. On shopping day, make sure you check expiration labels before you buy. And because changes in storage temperature can breed bacteria in many foods, shop for refrigerated and frozen foods last and make sure they're the first items to be put away when you get home.

All raw meat, poultry, and seafood should be double wrapped and stored in a separate area of your refrigerator to prevent any juices from contaminating other foods. These raw foods should also be isolated from other foods during meal preparation. Keep your refrigerator clean, and wipe up spills immediately when they occur to discourage bacteria growth.

When preparing raw meat, eggs, poultry, fish, or shellfish, immediately and thoroughly clean all knives, dishes, cutting boards, food prep surfaces, and utensils that have come in contact with the food before it is transferred to the stovetop or oven. And, of course, wash your hands—with hot, soapy water. Then get a clean set of utensils and serving dishes for use with the cooked food.

Fruits and veggies should also get a good cleaning. Thoroughly rinse everything you get from the produce stand and your own garden. Even veggies that are precut and packaged (for example, bagged salad greens, baby carrots) should be washed again before eating.

When cooking meat and poultry, make sure it's well done by using a meat thermometer. Cook ground beef and pork to an internal temperature of 160°F, well-done steaks to 170°F, and whole chicken to 180°F (chicken breasts need only to reach 170°F).

Finally, when it's time to put away the leftovers, make sure you seal them up tightly and immediately refrigerate them. Leftovers should be refrigerated within 2 hours.

Dining Out

You can't ensure safe handling and preparation of your meals when you're not in control of the kitchen. But treating yourself to the occasional night out at a restaurant is perhaps even more important now that you're pregnant. When possible, go to restaurants you know and trust. When dining someplace new, stick with safe menu choices that are less likely to harbor food-borne illness. Avoid anything sold off a cart or truck, and steer clear of eateries that look poorly kept and dirty (chances are the kitchen is, too).

When your meal is done, skip the doggie bag. Food should be refrigerated within 2 hours—counting from the moment the cook sticks it under the heat lamp. Allowing for a leisurely meal, a reasonably efficient wait staff, and travel time home from the restaurant, it's more than likely you won't make the cutoff—giving your leftovers time to incubate bacteria.

Alcohol—The Facts

So, what about alcohol? You may have heard that moderate consumption of a drink or two a week is safe in pregnancy. The truth is that there is no known safe level of alcohol intake in pregnancy, and it's unclear how much may have an impact on the development of your unborn child. Bottom line: Complete abstinence is the safest route for baby. That said, if you have had a cocktail since conception, perhaps before you even discovered you were pregnant, there is no point is obsessing over it. Letting the incident consume you with guilt or allowing it to become a source of undue stress is bad for you and baby. Instead, focus your energies on living a healthy lifestyle now.

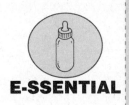

E-SSENTIAL

If you have a drinking or substance abuse problem, seeking help early in your pregnancy is imperative. Alcoholics Anonymous (A.A.) can be a source of steadfast support and inspiration. A.A. meetings are free of charge and easily accessible, with over 52,000 groups in the United States. Go online to *www.aa.org* or check your local telephone directory to find one in your area.

The consequences of continuing alcohol use during pregnancy range from risking miscarriage to causing an array of physical, mental, behavioral, and developmental problems known as *fetal alcohol spectrum disorders* (FASD). One of the most severe is fetal alcohol syndrome (FAS). Babies born with FAS experience growth retardation and central nervous system problems, as well as develop characteristic facial features including small eye openings, a small head, a short upturned nose, absence of the groove between the upper lip and the nose, and an undeveloped outer ear. FAS is permanent and irreversible.

Central nervous system (CNS) difficulties can prevent newborns from being able to suckle and can create conditions in children of tremulousness, hyperactivity, low IQ, behavioral problems, learning disabilities, and language delays. More specifically, alcohol consumption in the first trimester of pregnancy is responsible for the facial anomalies of FAS, while growth retardation, birth defects, and CNS problems can be triggered by drinking at any point in pregnancy. Children with only some of these symptoms (for example, CNS problems and growth retardation, but not facial anomalies) are classified as having fetal alcohol effects (FAE),

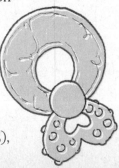

alcohol-related neurodevelopmental disabilities (ARND), or alcohol-related birth defects (ARBD).

Because the first 8 weeks of pregnancy are a time of rapid development for the limbs, heart, central nervous system, and other organ systems of the embryo, it's important now—before it's too late—to get a handle on even occasional drinking, not to mention binge or frequent drinking. Talk to your health care provider about treatment options, or turn to your church or local social service agency for support.

Month 4

Welcome to the second trimester—what many women consider "the fun part." Your energy is up, and your meals are staying down. Your pregnancy is now a visible fact, so indulge in the occasional daytime nap and take advantage of designated close-in pregnancy parking spaces without feeling guilty. You and your baby are headed into a period of rapid growth now, so hang on and enjoy the ride. Here's a look at what you can anticipate in month 4.

Baby This Month

Snoozing, stretching, swallowing, and even thumb sucking, your fetus is busy this month as he tests out his new reflexes and abilities. He is losing his top-heavy look as his height starts to catch up to his head size. By the end of this month, he will measure about 6 to 8 inches in length and weigh approximately 6 ounces.

Now is a good time to begin singing to, reading to, and even playing music for your little one. The inner ear structures that allow him to hear are developing this month. He has grown eyebrows, eyelashes, and possibly even a little hair on top.

The long bones of his arms and legs are growing, as cartilage is replaced with spongy, woven, soft bone in a process called *ossification*. Skeletal development will continue long after birth and well into adolescence and young adulthood.

Your baby is inhaling and exhaling amniotic fluid, practicing his technique for his first breath in the outside world. The lungs are already generating cellular fluid and a substance known as *surfactant*. In later months the surfactant will assist the development of the fetal lungs by expanding the alveoli (air sacs) within them. These substances move out through the trachea and become part of the amniotic fluid, along with the urine your unborn child is already passing.

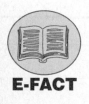

E-FACT

The umbilical cord contains two arteries and a vein sheathed with a gelatinous tissue known as Wharton's jelly. The jelly cushions the blood vessels and protects them from kinks and twists. Although umbilical cord knots do occur, they are relatively rare, happening in approximately 1 percent of pregnancies.

The placenta is approximately 3 inches in diameter this month; the attached umbilical cord is about as long as the fetus and continues to grow. Fetal blood is being pumped through this little body at about 4 miles an hour, exiting through the two large arteries in the umbilical cord and on to the placenta. In the placenta, baby's waste products (urine and carbon dioxide) are exchanged for oxygenated, nutrient-rich blood that is returned to the fetus via the umbilical cord vein. Pressure from the blood pumping within the cord helps straighten it out and keeps it from becoming knotted or getting in the way of your unborn baby's kicks and somersaults. Total time for this complex exchange? About 30 seconds.

Your Body This Month

In pregnancy, feeling is believing. Although hearing baby's heartbeat or seeing fetal movement on an ultrasound monitor are milestone moments, the first time you actually sense your child inside of you—proof positive that you are indeed nurturing an actual human being—is a humbling and life-affirming experience.

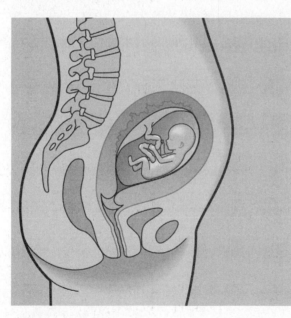

You and your fetus in the 4th month of pregnancy

Your Body Changes

If you weren't showing last month, chances are you will have a definite pregnant profile by the end of this month. Your uterus is about the size of a head of cabbage, and its top tip lies just below your bellybutton.

What You Feel Like

Your appetite may start to pick up this month, especially if you've been too sick to enjoy a good meal until now. You'll need a healthy craving or two to fuel fetal growth: About 60 percent of your total pregnancy weight (about 11 to 15 pounds) will be gained in this trimester.

E-FACT

The thin line of fine hair that runs from your navel down to your pubic bone—the *linea alba*—may turn dark in pregnancy, again thanks to hormonal changes. If you do develop this little stripe, now called a *linea nigra*, it will most likely lighten again postpartum.

Heartburn may start to become a persistent problem as your uterus crowds your stomach and the smooth muscles of your digestive tract remain relaxed due to the hormone progesterone. Some tips for putting out the fire:

✓ Avoid greasy, fatty, and spicy foods.

✓ Stay away from alcohol and caffeinated drinks (for example, cola, tea, coffee); these can relax the valve between the stomach and the esophagus and exacerbate heartburn.

✓ Keep a food log to determine your heartburn triggers.

✓ Eat smaller, more frequent meals instead of three large ones.

✓ Drink plenty of water between meals to reduce stomach acid.

✓ Don't eat just before you go to bed or lie down to rest.

✓ Rest your head on a few extra pillows in bed to assist gravity in easing heartburn while you sleep.

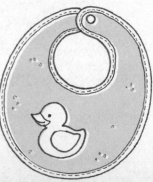

If heartburn symptoms won't relent, there are several over-the-counter antacids and medications available that are considered safe to use in pregnancy. Speak with your doctor to find out which one may be right for you.

E-ALERT!

Calcium—it does a baby good. Your little one needs lots of calcium to build bone and blood cells and regulate heart rhythm. Milk is an excellent source; 3½ cups each day provide you with the recommended 1,000 milligrams. If you're under age nineteen, you should have an additional 300 mg daily. Yogurt, broccoli, kale, and salmon are rich in calcium as well.

As if heartburn weren't enough to deal with, pregnancy might start to become a real pain in the rear, literally. Many women develop hemorrhoids, which are caused by increased pressure on the rectal veins. Your growing uterus places pressure on the inferior vena cava, the vein that services the lower body, while pregnancy hormones cause veins to dilate (widen), encouraging swelling. And by straining to have a bowel movement, you may put undue stress on the rectal veins, which can become blocked—trapping blood, turning itchy and painful, and perhaps even protruding from the anus. Exercise, a high-fiber diet, and plenty of water can help to avoid constipation and straining with bowel movements that may aggravate the condition. Try easing the pain with an ice pack, a soak in a warm tub, wipes with witch hazel pads, or a topical prescription cream as recommended by your doctor.

Hemorrhoids do have the potential to become more than just a minor discomfort, so be sure to speak with your provider if they do occur. Although they typically resolve after pregnancy, in some cases clotting occurs and surgery is necessary.

Other symptoms of second-trimester pregnancy that you may start or continue to experience this month include:

✓ Nausea
✓ Fatigue
✓ Frequent urination

- ✓ Tender and/or swollen breasts
- ✓ Bleeding gums
- ✓ Excess mucus and saliva
- ✓ Increase in normal vaginal discharge
- ✓ Mild shortness of breath
- ✓ Lightheadedness or dizziness
- ✓ Gas and/or constipation
- ✓ Skin and hair changes
- ✓ Feeling warm or easily overheated

Movement!

Think that ultrasound was exciting? Just wait until you feel your little gymnast stretch and push inside of you for the first time. If this is your second or third child, you may already recognize the familiar sensation of her little body flexing in your slightly used womb. For moms in their debut pregnancy with somewhat less stretchy accommodations, the first movements (known as *quickening*) may not be felt quite as early. But by week 19, most women have felt that distinctive first flutter.

So, what does it feel like? It's often described in terms of butterfly wings or bubbles or, less poetically, as gas or a block of jiggling JELL-O in the abdomen. Because pregnancy can cause so many gastrointestinal symptoms, you might not even notice the gentle nudges of baby until he's been persistent with his movements for a few days.

You'll quickly discover that your baby is already establishing behavioral patterns. When you're up and about, he can be rocked to sleep by your movements. Then when you lie down and try to take a rest, he wants to get up and groove. Is your partner having trouble getting a hand on your stomach in time to feel the fetal kung fu? Have him stand by during a lying-down time and see whether he catches a kick or two.

Once baby starts moving regularly, the sensation quickly becomes second nature. On average, you should feel five or more movements each hour from your passenger. Three or fewer movements or a sudden decrease in fetal activity could be a sign of fetal distress, so if you notice either, call your provider to follow up as soon as possible.

The Shape You're In

Carrying high or low? Looking large—or barely showing? It's practically inevitable that at some point in your pregnancy someone will try to guess the gender of your child based on how your belly is filled out. Although guessing is an entertaining way to pass the time, the theory that high means a girl and low means a boy has no basis in science. How you carry is dependent on your build, posture, and pregnancy history. Women who have had a previous pregnancy tend to have more pliable abdominal muscles and therefore often carry lower. The baby's position also influences your pregnant topography, which may change from one day to the next.

At Your Doctor Visit

If you didn't listen to the fetal heartbeat last month, you'll likely get your chance with this visit. Women who have chosen to take an AFP/triple/quad test will have their blood drawn sometime between week 15 and week 18.

On Your Mind

You're now hitting your stride as the wooziness and uncertainties of the first 3 months fade away and the discomforts of late pregnancy still lie relatively far ahead.

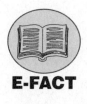

E-FACT

Varicella infection (chickenpox) can cause serious complications in pregnancy. If you have never had chickenpox or the vaccine and are exposed to the virus, contact your health care provider immediately. If your blood tests negative for varicella antibodies, immediate treatment with varicella-zoster immune globulin (VZIG) can prevent or lessen the severity of chickenpox.

Feeling better and having more energy, you might be ready to conquer the world (or at least the nursery). Yet coworkers, friends, and family now starting to recognize you as "a pregnant woman" may be handling you with kid gloves.

The pampering is nice, within limits. Accept the small favors that ease the discomforts of pregnancy—such as a closer parking space or the cushy chair in the conference room. But don't hesitate to be firm with those who pressure you to cut back on tasks you're perfectly capable of handling or who treat you like a porcelain doll.

Reality Strikes

For many women, the starter's pistol on motherhood goes off right when they feel baby's first pokes and prods. The palpable presence of your unborn child can trigger a series of mothering emotions—protectiveness, nurturing, nesting, and total impatience with anyone who poses a threat to the well-being of you and your child.

This maternal defense system might seem a bit extreme to the husband who is banished from the bedroom when he has a head cold, or the visiting friend who is asked to take his cigarette outside in subzero weather, but you aren't being paranoid or unreasonable. No one would think twice about keeping a newborn away from sneezing and smoking; a developing fetus is just as vulnerable, if not more so.

Exercise

Don't avoid the gym, pool, or other favorite fitness hangouts just because you're pregnant. Exercise will not only make you feel better; it can also tone muscles that will be getting a workout in labor and delivery. Feeling alarmingly large among the gym babes? Try mixing up your routine with something new like hiking, golf (sans cart), or a prenatal exercise class.

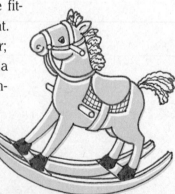

So, how much exercise is too much? It depends upon your prepregnancy fitness level. If you were swimming an hour each day before pregnancy, there's no reason not to continue that routine if you have your provider's blessing. On the other hand, don't start training for a marathon if your notion of exercise is walking into McDonald's instead of using the drive-thru. The rule of thumb for women in pregnancies that are not high-risk is that 30 minutes of moderate exercise daily is ideal.

E-QUESTION

Are my vivid dreams related to pregnancy?
Dreams that are exceptionally vivid, disturbing, or just plain bizarre are common in pregnancy. Your dreams are reflections of what's on your mind, so it's natural for them to feature the baby, your family, and the future. They can seem larger than life right now due to insecurities about the future and those pregnancy hormones.

Benefits

If you weren't into a regular fitness routine before pregnancy, exercise could be the least appealing thing you can imagine right now. Try to set your distaste aside for a few moments and consider the benefits a regular workout provides:

✓ **Energy up.** Stretching and moving daily boosts your energy level and calms your mind.

✓ **Postpartum weight down.** It will be easier to work off your pregnancy weight after the birth if you already have a regular routine.

✓ **Ease your aches and pains.** Exercise that promotes strength and flexibility can prevent or diminish lower-back pain, muscle-aches, and other complaints of pregnancy.

✓ **Positive mental attitude.** Feeling fit can improve your self-image.

Staying Active

Exercise doesn't have to be complicated, expensive, or technically difficult. It can be as simple as tossing a ball with the kids in the backyard, taking the dog on a brisk walk each evening, or swimming or even walking laps in the local pool. Thirty minutes of regular, heart-pumping activity, started and capped off with a good stretching routine, is all it takes to benefit you and baby. Above all, make sure it's an activity you enjoy or do in good company so that you will look forward to it.

E-ALERT!

Certain activities are definitely off-limits during pregnancy. These include scuba diving, water skiing, and contact sports. In addition, proceed with caution when participating in potentially high-impact activities like tennis, volleyball, and aerobics. As always, run any new or prepregnancy fitness routine by your health care provider before you take part.

If you thrive on routine and feel more likely to get moving if you have a set schedule, check out your local YMCA, hospital, or community center for a prenatal exercise class. Water exercise programs are also a good low-impact way to get fit. Even if your class is tailored toward moms-to-be, check with your doctor first.

Precautions

While exercise can be a boon to your body and baby, there are basic steps you should take to stay safe. First and foremost, run your routine by your provider to get a medical stamp of approval. If you're new to working out, start slowly. Be attuned to your body's signals and stop immediately if you experience warning signs such as abdominal or chest pain, vaginal bleeding, dizziness, blurred vision, severe headache, or excessive shortness of breath.

Dress in supportive, comfortable clothing that breathes well and braces your belly and other parts of your expanding anatomy. If your feet have swollen past the comfort level of your old gym shoes, invest in a bigger pair. Drink plenty of caffeine-free fluids before, during, and after your workout to remain well-hydrated, and try to work out in a climate-controlled environment to avoid a sharp rise in core body temperature, because overheating can be hazardous to a developing fetus.

Kegels are one exercise every pregnant woman should know and practice. They strengthen the pelvic muscles for delivery and can improve the urinary incontinence (dribbling) that some women experience in pregnancy. What's a Kegel? Tighten the muscles you use to shut off your urine flow, hold for 4 seconds, and relax. You've just done your first Kegel. Try to work up to 10 minutes of Kegels daily.

Just for Dads

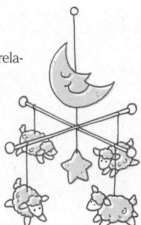

Every couple bickers once in a while. In fact, many relationships seem to thrive on heated debate. But the hormonal tidal wave and stressors that accompany pregnancy can bring an unexpected addition of friction to the mix. Try to remain sensitive to your partner's physical and mental changes without being condescending. In other words, "Honey, I know it's just the hormones talking" is not a good way to resolve an argument.

Understanding Her Emotions

You can't feel her aches and pains, but you can feel the brunt of her volatile emotions. Even if you understand why she's moody, with all this exposed emotional wiring, you might be tempted to keep a low profile. Remember, your partner needs empathy and assistance right now, not professions of sympathy and avoidance. Support her with your actions, love, and acceptance, and you can make it through this pregnancy with an even stronger bond.

You may be starting to feel the "But what about me?" syndrome coming on. The hullabaloo surrounding your significant other and your unborn child might be making you feel a little (maybe even very) neglected. Your partner is focusing on the pregnancy and baby instead of you. Feeling left out or even jealous is perfectly normal. Try to address your feelings by arranging some special couple time for your partner and you, when you both can be waited on and pampered a bit. Splurge on a night out at a special restaurant, a weekend at a nice hotel, or a double massage. And also keep in mind that as father-to-be you have a special role to play in this pregnancy; both mom and baby are relying on your support, coaching, patience, and love.

What You Can Do to Help

Be patient. You will be expected to use your mind-reading capabilities to their fullest extent. In other words, your partner may not ask for help, but you need to offer it (and offer it frequently). Then follow through soon after without procrastinating. If she is in nesting mode, chances are she won't let things sit undone for long. If you don't follow through, then all you've done is compound her stress with irritation.

Volunteer for errands and chores that are starting to become physically difficult for her pregnant body, such as weekly trips to the Laundromat, mowing the lawn, and taking your ill-behaved St. Bernard to the groomer. Let her sleep in on the weekends. Take care of some of those household repair tasks you've been meaning to get to before she has to remind you about them.

If you already have other children, it's easy to let your partner's rest and mental health needs take a back seat as other parental responsibilities come to the forefront. Consider getting some extra help around the house from relatives or even a biweekly cleaning service to keep daily life manageable.

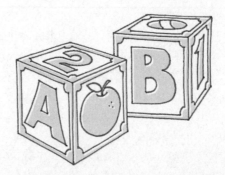

Working During Pregnancy

Pregnancy is a great time to take a step back and re-assess where you are, and where you're headed, on your career path. Take the opportunity to align your professional goals with the new challenges of parenting. You might be anxious about functioning well on the job during your pregnancy. Recognize your value as an employee and as a woman. Don't let anyone make you feel guilty about being pregnant. Know your legal rights, stick to your guns, and realize you don't have to settle for the status quo when it comes to the workplace.

Your Rights

Unfortunately, it's sometimes easier to change the legal structures of the employment landscape than alter prevalent workplace attitudes and prejudices. Too frequently, pregnancy is construed as a personal indication that you have no need for professional fulfillment.

Even if you do consider work nothing more than a way to pay the bills, your rights are still important. Intolerant and illegal practices concerning pregnancy in the workplace can result in financial loss as career advancement screeches to a halt, you get the minimum salary bump at your next annual review, and bigger and better job offers dry up. Fortunately, federal and state statutes are in place to minimize the chances that you will be professionally or economically punished for your choice to become a mother.

The Pregnancy Discrimination Act

The Pregnancy Discrimination Act is a 1978 amendment to Title VII of the Civil Rights Act of 1964. The act requires that your employer provide you with the same rights, resources, accommodations, and benefits as other employees who are on temporary disability due to illness or injury. It also dictates that your employer must allow you to work as long as you are physically able to do your job. Keep in mind that the act only applies to businesses with more than fifteen employees; and, if your employer does not provide disability benefits to injured or ill employees, there will be no benefits for your pregnancy either.

E-FACT

If you belong to a union, talk to your union representative about maternity and paternity leave under your contract. You may have additional rights and benefits that aren't available to nonunion employees at your workplace, and in some cases these can exceed the benefits covered by state and federal law.

If you're searching for a new position while pregnant, the Pregnancy Discrimination Act protects you from prejudice on the basis of your pregnancy. Still, legalities aside, pregnancy may make your interviewer look for other viable reasons not to hire you. It's illegal for a potential employer to ask if you're pregnant or not in the interview, and you certainly aren't required to volunteer the information. However, if the job is offered to you, it is probably in your best interest to mention your pregnancy during final negotiations. You want to start your working relationship off on the right foot and address up front any concerns your prospective employer has.

The Family and Medical Leave Act (FMLA)

If you or your spouse works for a public agency, a private or public elementary or secondary school, or a company with more than fifty employees for a period of at least a year, you have coverage under the Family and Medical Leave Act (FMLA). The FMLA provides for up to 12 weeks of unpaid leave within a 12-month period for medical and family caretaking reasons, including the care of a newborn child. Both moms and dads are eligible as long as they meet the employment criteria.

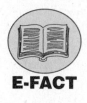

E-FACT

New parents who have been denied FMLA leave from their employer and believe they are eligible can file a complaint with the U.S. Department of Labor (DOL). The complaint must be filed within 2 years of the incident. Call the DOL at 1-866-4USWAGE for further information.

The FMLA also enables you to take unpaid time off if you experience health problems during pregnancy and your employer does not provide disability or sick-day benefits. The same goes for extended time off that you might require to care for your child should she have any health problems at birth. Again, the total time off provided for under the FMLA is not to exceed a total of 12 weeks in 12 months.

State Law

Depending on where you live, your state may mandate certain employee rights related to pregnancy and maternity benefits under workers' compensation laws. Check with the labor department or other applicable organization in your state to find out more.

Occupational Hazards

Depending on your position and work environment, you might have to alter your duties temporarily or request a change in location or accommodations. If your job involves any of the following conditions, talk with your human resources department about your options:

- **Weight lifting.** Lifting heavy packages, boxes, or other items (for example, shipping and receiving clerks, warehouse work) is not recommended in pregnancy, especially past week 20.
- **Secondhand smoke.** Women who work in the hospitality industry (for example, bartenders, waitresses) expose their fetuses to toxins in secondhand smoke.
- **High heat.** Excessive temperatures (for example, summer construction, factory environment) can be harmful to fetal development, particularly in the first trimester.
- **Teratogen exposure.** Jobs that involve working with certain chemicals and hazardous substances (for example, welders and lead exposure, dry cleaners and benzene exposure) are linked to birth defects.
- **Standing and repetitive movement.** Line work or other jobs that keep you on your feet all day (for example, factory jobs, assembly work, piece work) can exacerbate circulatory problems.
- **Ionizing radiation exposure.** Pregnant pilots and flight crew may be exposed to excessive ionizing radiation, another known teratogen. Radiographic imaging technicians who work with x-rays, CT scanning equipment, and nuclear medicine are also at risk.

Breaking the News

In an ideal world, the news of your impending motherhood would be greeted with congratulations and reassurances at the office. Instead, reality may find you strategizing to prevent a negative employer reaction and determining the right time to drop the pregnancy bombshell for minimal fallout to your career. That pregnancy should be considered a handicap to be overcome rather than the positive, life-affirming force it is remains a glaring reminder of how far women still have to go to achieve equality in the workplace.

E-ALERT!

According to the American Academy of Family Physicians (AAFP), the maximum safe fetal radiation dose during pregnancy is 5 rad. If you require x-rays or other radiological tests during pregnancy, the benefits of imaging need to be weighed against the potential risk to the fetus. If at all possible, tests involving radiation should be avoided during pregnancy. If the test is needed, however, radiology staff will do everything possible to minimize your exposure.

When you do inform your employer, make sure he hears it directly from you and not by way of the water cooler. Accompany the news with your tentative schedule for maternity leave so that your manager can plan accordingly. Offering suggestions for a replacement in your absence or ways to temporarily reassign workload will reflect well on you and your perceived commitment to your employer.

Avoiding the "Mommy Track" Trap

Once you share your news, you may suddenly find yourself on a slow road to nowhere at work—last in the information loop and out of the running for promotions and job advancements you were previously an easy pick for. Goodbye fast track and hello mommy track? Is it unavoidable?

Not necessarily. Employers who realize that a happy employee is more likely to be a productive employee won't punish you for pursuing a personal life. And if you continue to perform well and make it clear to your supervisors that you'd like to have a career path with the company rather than just a job, you're more likely to avoid the so-called "mommy track." Still, whether the mommy track exists in your organization or not depends on the corporate culture and the attitudes of upper management. Do they support family-friendly policies? Do they lead by example and make use of benefits like paternity and maternity leave themselves? And are efforts made to institute initiatives that benefit employees across the board, from the security staff to the CEO?

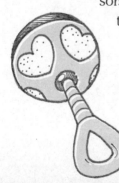

The Ideal Versus the Real

In the real world, some organizations reward those who invest themselves more fully in the workplace than in family. The result is an atmosphere in which pregnancy is construed as a choice against company and career, a choice that may be tolerated for the sake of political correctness but that certainly isn't supported through policies and reward systems. The good news is that there are family-friendly employers who put their benefits packages where their mouth is. See where your company lies between these two extremes:

The ideal . . . a fully equipped lactation facility.
The real . . . a bathroom stall with a broken lock.

The ideal . . . paid time off for prenatal appointments.
The real . . . isn't that what lunch hours are for?

The ideal . . . expectant-mother parking spaces near the entrance.
The real . . . unless you are a VIP, it's first come, first served.

The ideal . . . a pregnant supervisor to commiserate with.
The real . . . your bachelor boss is a freshly minted MBA who thinks "family-friendly policy" means Christmas off with pay.

The ideal . . . a flexible schedule for your unpredictable pregnant body.
The real . . . don't forget to punch out for bathroom breaks.

The ideal . . . 4 months of maternity leave with full pay and benefits.
The real . . . with luck, that partial disability pay should arrive before your child's first birthday.

Defining Personal and Professional Goals

What do you want out of life, both personally and professionally, now that your family is changing? If this is your first child, it can be hard to fully assess the new direction you're taking. But there are probably some basic decisions you can make with a degree of certainty. For example, late shifts and working double overtime may be out of the picture for you now.

If you work in an environment that isn't healthy for you or your growing baby, talk to your human resources department about a temporary reassignment to a more appropriate position. Jobs that involve chemical exposure, heavy manual labor, or staying on your feet all day with no opportunity for rest should all be reconsidered during pregnancy.

Perhaps you have career goals that you'd like to keep on target. Should they be mutually exclusive of motherhood? No. Might they be, depending on where you work? Yes. If you wanted to move into a supervisory position at your next review but see your company promoting only those who work excessive overtime, you have choices to make. Such is the delicate balance of motherhood. Fortunately, you always have the option to look for a workplace that is more in harmony with your personal and professional goals—or to take your own path, whatever it may be.

Realize Your Value

Think of full-time motherhood as another job offer on the table for your employer to stack up to. Your company could be willing to sweeten the pot with flextime, telecommuting, or other family-friendly working arrangements to keep you happy. Remember, in most cases it has poured a significant amount of money and resources into your training. The loss of that investment plus the cost of hiring and training a new employee is a big financial incentive for keeping you on board. Don't be afraid to rock the boat. Realize your value and use it as a bargaining chip.

Negotiate Toward Your Goal

Think about using your maternity leave as a launching pad for alternative working arrangements. For example, if you would like more than the 6 weeks of paid leave your company offers and would ultimately like some flexibility in your schedule, suggest a work arrangement like telecommuting for another 6 weeks following paid leave. If you're covered by the FMLA, your employer must give you 12 weeks off without pay to care for your newborn, if you request it. By offering an alternative to your complete absence, you appear flexible and dedicated, and your employer certainly has nothing to lose by trying such an arrangement. Even if you aren't prepared to take 6 weeks off unpaid should your employer turn you down, it's well worth the gamble to suggest the idea. You can always scale back your plans if your request isn't granted. And if it is accepted and works out well, you will have proven yourself for handling a more permanent arrangement down the road.

Practical Matters

No matter what your job, staying comfortable, relatively stressless, and economically secure during your pregnancy is essential.

Staying Comfortable

Pregnant women who do work on their feet should make a habit of changing positions often and moving when possible. Wear comfortable shoes and consider support stockings.

For jobs that require a lot of sit-down time, make sure you have an ergonomically appropriate chair that promotes good posture. A lumbar support pad can help ease pregnancy-related lower-back pain, and you can put up your feet under your desk on a small stool or even on a stack of phone books. If you work a desk job, look for opportunities to get up and about. Take a walk to speak with a coworker instead of picking up the phone, or hand-deliver a memo instead of using e-mail.

Scheduling Doctor Visits

With luck, your employer recognizes that good prenatal care translates to a healthier, more productive employee and, in the long run, to less time spent out of the office to care for sick kids. However, if you do face resistance in taking time off for doctor visits, remember that prenatal care is considered necessary medical care and is covered under the FMLA. If all else fails, you can invoke your legal rights.

In the meantime, find out whether your provider has evening, weekend, or early morning appointments that might fit around your workday. If you must go during office hours and your supervisor isn't pleased, offer her the alternative option of taking the entire day off as vacation or unpaid leave instead. Perhaps she'll look upon your short absence in a new light.

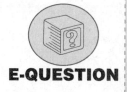

E-QUESTION

I asked for three months of unpaid maternity leave and was fired for a "lack of dedication." What can I do?
Contact the U.S. Equal Employment Opportunity Commission (EEOC) office at 1-800-669-4000. If you're covered by the FMLA, your former employer has broken the law. Don't wait too long; there are time limits on when charges of employment discrimination must be filed.

If you're getting static for meeting basic prenatal care requirements now, just think what it will be like when you need time off to care for a sick child or to keep a well-baby appointment. File a mental note: family unfriendly. Companies that score poorly in supporting their pregnant employees will probably continue the trend postpregnancy. If too many red flags are raised during your pregnancy, once you reach maternity leave it's probably time to look for a company that recognizes the value of personal as well as professional fulfillment in their employees.

Controlling Stress

The workplace can be a stress hotbed. Deadlines, personality conflicts, difficult clients, quotas, overtime, and more make for a pressure cooker that's not good for you or baby. Try to maintain some perspective and peace of mind by realizing that petty office politics means little in comparison to the health and well-being of your child.

Remember that others don't control your feelings; you do. If work pressures and the attitudes of others are starting to wear you down, consider a yoga or meditation class to keep yourself balanced. And when possible, take a short mental health break during the work day to decompress. A regular lunchtime walk can help clear your mind and it's good exercise as well.

Maternity Leave

Your bonding time with baby should be free of workplace concerns. If you plan appropriately for your absence as early as possible, you'll get more out of your time off. It's a good idea to put all maternity leave plans in writing for your supervisor and appropriate managers and to make an extra copy for placement in your personnel file.

Planning Ahead for Leave

Lay the groundwork for your maternity leave so that there won't be too many questions or crises in your absence. If appropriate for your position, delegate some tasks to coworkers and arrange coverage by others. Find out if your supervisor plans on hiring temporary help to fill in during your absence, and prepare training materials and checklists so that you won't face a mess upon your return to the workplace.

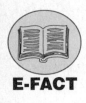

E-FACT

According to a 2010 benefits survey performed by the Society for Human Resource Management, paid paternity leave was offered by only 17 percent of companies polled. If your workplace doesn't offer paid paternity leave, dads may qualify for unpaid time off under the Family Medical Leave Act.

Check and double-check that all appropriate paperwork for benefits has been filled out, signed, and sent in well in advance of your planned departure. Maternity leave should be a low-stress time, not one that requires twice-weekly contact with human resources to find out the status of your disability claim.

How Many Weeks?

So, just how much, or how little, maternity leave should you take? Certainly the benefits your company provides will play a major factor in your decision. If you have quite a bit of seniority, you may be able to swing an even longer leave by tapping into accrued vacation time. Other factors to consider include:

✓ **Money.** How much time off can you afford if your maternity benefits are minimal or nonexistent? Don't forget to factor into your equation any money you'll be saving (that is, dry cleaning bills, lunches out, transportation expenses) by not working.

✓ **Management.** Even though you may be legally within your rights, in some organizations an extended maternity leave may be frowned upon by those above you. Consider what management might think and, more importantly, what kind of priority you should place on their disapproval.

✓ **Morale.** Are your coworkers and/or subordinates happy and motivated or disillusioned and resentful? Employees who work as a team and feel invested in their workplace are more likely to rise to the challenge in your absence.

✓ **Malleability.** Does employment have to be all or nothing? Think about offering some creative proposals for extending your leave, such as a reduced part-time schedule or the prospect of telecommuting.

Evaluating your leave options will reveal the pluses and negatives in your company's attitudes toward personal employee fulfillment. If morale is poor and management unyielding, once you've gotten past maternity leave it may be time to consider your work alternatives.

Back to Work

After you deliver your child, the toughest day you'll have is that first time back to work. You'll worry about whether his caregiver will be able to tell his hungry cry from his tired cry, whether he's getting the attention he thrives on, and (of course) whether he misses you. Try to focus on the benefits of the situation—the increased value of the time you and your baby do have together,

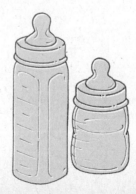

his broadening horizons as he interacts with new children and adults, and the financial security your family is gaining.

Easing the Transition

No matter how you slice it, it will be hard being away from your baby. If you can, start back on a part-time arrangement to ease into the separation. Drop in at day care during your lunch hour if logistically possible. Above all, make the most of the time you do have together with your child by making home a work-free zone.

Striking a Balance

In your premommy life, you may have set up certain expectations that you find yourself hard pressed to live up to now. It's time to redefine appropriate work limits, even if it means setting new boundaries. Coworkers and clients who felt free to contact you before via cell phones, texting, and instant messaging, day or night, now need to be gently guided to restricting contact to the office or at least re-evaluating the urgency of their issues before trying to reach you. Getting some control back over your time might be as simple as gradually ridding yourself of all the extra gadgetry that makes you painfully accessible and encouraging your colleagues to leave you a voice mail or send an e-mail.

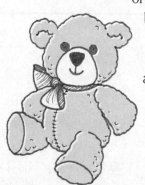

Women who work nontraditional schedules can have special needs for achieving balance. Evening "day care" can be tough to find without friends or relatives in the area, and schedules that change on a weekly basis can make child care even more difficult to plan on. Talk to your supervisor candidly about your needs and see whether a shift change or a more permanent schedule can be arranged. If you're a dependable and valued employee, your employer would rather work with you to retain your skills and experience.

Changing Paths

A corporate culture that was perfect for your childless lifestyle may not fit your new family way of living. If the nature of your job or employer makes it impossible for you to achieve that delicate work/home balance, it's probably time to change direction with a new employer.

Family-Friendly Companies: What to Look For

Few organizations will admit to being family unfriendly when questioned during the interview process. Uncovering the truth will take some detective work on your part.

Finding out about flextime options when you're in the process of interviewing can be a sticky situation. In many organizations, arrangements like telecommuting are still reserved as a privilege for those who have proven their value to the company. Unless the job description includes flexible working arrangements, you're better off not inquiring directly about the possibility. Instead ask broad questions about available benefits and the average workday, which will reveal the information in due course.

You can look to resources like business-focused local and national media as a starting point. (Both *Fortune* and *Working Mother* magazines put out an annual "100 Best Companies to Work For" list.) Corporate annual reports can also be a good source of information. Once your foot is in the door and you're going through the interview process, make sure you have an opportunity to talk to potential coworkers to get an overview of available benefits and programs. A few programs and plans that are good indications a company is family friendly include:

✓ **Flexibility.** Does the company have written policies on options like flextime, job sharing, and telecommuting?

✓ **Lactation facilities.** Are there comfortable areas dedicated to breast-feeding or breastmilk pumping? If not, is your employer willing to provide an appropriate private space?

✓ **Paid paternity leave.** Are dads given time off for a new baby, either with pay or at least without prejudice? If a policy is in place, is it used successfully?

✓ **On-site child care or child care assistance.** If your workplace doesn't have on-site or sponsored child care, does it offer enrollment in a flexible spending account that allows you to save up to $5,000 tax free to pay child care expenses?

✓ **Time-saving perks.** These run the gamut from on-site dry cleaning and retail services to employee concierge services that can run small errands for you.

✓ **Value placed on education.** Corporate-sponsored scholarships for children of employees, tuition assistance, and mentorship programs with local schools are a few ways a company can express how it values education.

Flextime, Telecommuting, and Other Options

Even if your company doesn't have established flexible working options, it can't hurt to pitch such an idea to your supervisor or to the human resources department. There's always a first, and you would be blazing the trail for others who follow.

Realize, however, that your job position needs to be conducive to the arrangement you're suggesting. If you have a computer-intensive desk job that could be performed remotely, you're more likely to get a telecommuting arrangement than a receptionist whose job description requires a physical presence. Consider what type of flexible arrangement your position would work with. For example, a job-sharing arrangement might be perfect for the receptionist position.

Create a proposal that is well-researched and realistic. Outline in specific terms what you want out of the arrangement, including hours and logistical requirements (such as home computer equipment). Cover your contingencies, such as your availability for on-site meetings even when you aren't scheduled to be at the office.

Make sure you note the potential benefits to your employer as well. If office space is at a premium in your building, for example, a telecommuting arrangement will free up your desk for other employees. If your employer has no track record of flexible scheduling, the resulting boost in employee morale and company image can be a reputation enhancement.

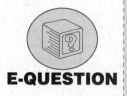
Just asking about flexible working options signals your willingness to consider greener pastures without an accommodation of your needs. If that happens, your employer loses time, talent, and money—three valuables that corporate America wants to grow, not squander. Make it easy for your company to say yes by putting together a well-considered and realistic proposal.

Full-Time at Home

Becoming a full-time mom is an exciting new venture for many women. If you can afford to stay home without working for someone else, go for it. Pouring your skills and knowledge into parenthood can be enormously fulfilling and in fact is probably the most rewarding job you'll ever have.

Finally, consider the possibility of forging your own family-friendly path. In today's wired world, many occupations lend themselves to home-based work; writing, income tax preparation, desktop publishing, and web design are naturals. If the field you currently work in is unfulfilling and you'd like to make a change, look to the hobbies you enjoy for some ideas. Refinishing antiques, creating crafts for retail, sewing, and painting are a few activities that might be a good fit for a new career. Starting something new is never easy, but just experiencing the miracle of your developing child can help you envision widening possibilities.

Month 5

You're still experiencing the relative comfort of the second trimester, but the aches and pains of pregnancy are starting to set in. Take heart; you're halfway there! Your energy and initiative are perhaps dampened by the dwindling quality of your sleep. Sleep deprivation can contribute to mental fuzziness and emotional edginess. If you haven't already, start to value and prioritize time spent between the sheets (asleep, that is).

Baby This Month

At 10 to 12 inches long and around 1 pound in weight, your baby is about the size of a regulation NFL football. How appropriate, considering you've reached the halftime of pregnancy.

Your little linebacker is starting to bulk up a bit as she accumulates deposits of brown fat under her skin. This insulation will help regulate her body temperature in the outside world. She's using her bulk to make her presence known; if you weren't feeling her last month, you likely are now. A look at her through ultrasound might reveal a wave of her clenched hands, which open and close freely now and have their own unique fingerprints.

The fetus is now covered in an oily white substance known as *vernix caseosa*, a sort of full-body fetal ChapStick that keeps her fluid-soaked skin from peeling and protects against infection. Some of the vernix will remain on the baby at birth, particularly in the skin folds (more if she is early, less if she is post-term).

Your Body This Month

As baby grows, your muscles and ligaments stretch to support this new weight. The result can be a new set of aches and pains as your body adjusts to the load.

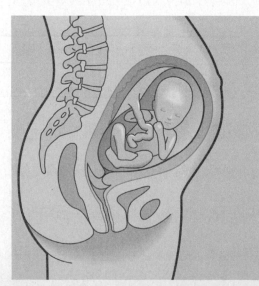

You and your baby halfway to the end zone

Your Body Changes

Feeling like you're turning inside out? Your "innie" may have already become an "outtie" as the skin of your belly (and accompanying button) is stretching, tightening, and most likely itching like crazy. A good moisturizing cream can relieve the itching and keep your skin hydrated, although it won't prevent or eliminate *striae gravidarum* (stretch marks). Whether you develop stretch marks is largely a matter of genetics, although factors such as excessive weight gain and multiples' gestations increase your odds of having them.

E-QUESTION

I think I'm getting varicose veins! What can I do to stop the discomfort?
Increased blood volume in pregnancy can damage the valves that regulate blood flow up through the blood vessels of the legs. The result is pooled blood in the vein and that telltale squiggly red or blue line. Supportive stockings and resting on your left side can relieve any leg soreness.

The red, purple, or whitish striae are created by the excess collagen your body produces in response to rapid stretching of the skin. They may appear on your abdomen, breasts, or on any other blossoming body part right now. Don't be too alarmed; striae typically fade to virtually invisible silver lines after pregnancy. If you do feel self-conscious, there are options for postpartum treatment of severe cases.

What You Feel Like

The band of ligaments supporting your uterus is carrying an increasingly heavy load. You might start to feel occasional discomfort in your lower abdomen, inner thighs, and hips, called *round ligament pain*. Pelvic tilt exercises are useful for keeping pelvic muscles toned and for relieving pain.

The pelvic tilt can be performed while standing against a wall, although it might be more comfortable done on your hands and knees following these steps: Keep your head aligned with your spine, pull in your abdomen, tighten your buttocks, and tilt the bottom of your pelvis forward. Your back will naturally arch up. Hold the position for 3 seconds, then relax. Remember to keep your back straight in this neutral position. Repeat the tilt 3 to 5 times, eventually working up to 10 repetitions.

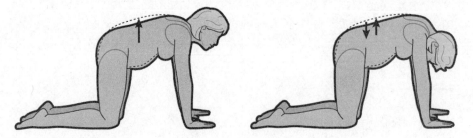

Pelvic tilts can tone your perineum and ease pregnancy aches and pains

Pregnancy hormones, the root of discomfort, are also contributing to the lower-back pain you could be experiencing. Progesterone and relaxin, the hormone responsible for softening your pelvic ligaments for delivery, are also loosening up your lower-back ligaments and disks; combined with the weight of your growing belly, your back is feeling the strain. Women who are having twins or more are especially prone to lower-back pain, which occurs in up to 50 percent of all pregnant women.

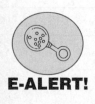

E-ALERT!

If your abdominal and/or back pains are severe or accompanied by fever, vomiting, vaginal bleeding, or leg numbness, call your health care provider immediately. Most minor back pain in pregnancy is completely normal, but in severe cases it can also be a sign of preterm labor, kidney infection, or other medical problems.

A few tips to help you ease your aches and pains:

✓ **Stand tall.** Perfect posture can go a long way toward easing back pain. Don't lead with your belly. Try to keep your center of gravity in your spine and pelvis. Check yourself by contracting your abdomen and buttock muscles at the same time, which should align your posture perfectly. Keep your head straight and your chin level. Your ears, shoulders, and hips should all be aligned.

✓ **Sit up straight.** Use good posture when you're sitting as well, and choose a chair with good lower-back support. You can purchase a special ergonomic support pad for your chair back, but a small pillow can do the trick just as easily.

✓ **Avoid twists and turns.** With your back so loose, a sudden move as simple as quickly turning at the waist to get out of bed may strain your back. Use your arms as support for a slow takeoff when rising from a chair.

✓ **Practice your pickups.** If you have small children who still need to be lifted occasionally, it's essential to use correct form. To avoid injury, bend and use your leg muscles to lift weight rather than bending from the waist and lifting with your back.

✓ **Warm up.** A warm pad on your back, hips, or other sore spots can help relieve pain.

✓ **Sensible shoes.** Avoid high heels! They will place further stress on your spine, and they're anything but comfy these days.

✓ **Foot rest.** Use a low stool or step to rest your feet when sitting. If you must stand for long periods, alternate resting each foot on a step.

✓ **Massage.** You now have a medical excuse to indulge in a regular back rub from your significant other. A licensed massage therapist who is experienced in prenatal massage would also be helpful.

✓ **Fluff and stuff.** Sleep on your side with a pillow placed between your legs. This will align your spine and improve your sleeping posture. A full-size body pillow can help support your back as well as belly.

✓ **Exercise.** If you aren't doing them already, some stretching and flexibility exercises may be in order. Check with your health care provider for approval and recommendations; if the pain is troublesome enough or if you have a history of back problems, she may suggest a physical therapist to work with.

Feeling hot and bothered? Pregnancy-induced changes in your metabolism and added weight can have you cranking the AC. Dress comfortably, cool off in the shower or tub, and invest in an extra fan if you don't have air conditioning.

Other symptoms that you may start or continue to experience this month include:

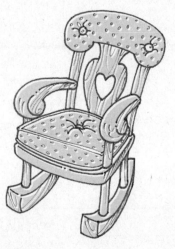

✓ Nausea
✓ Fatigue
✓ Frequent urination
✓ Tender and/or swollen breasts
✓ Bleeding gums
✓ Excess mucus and saliva
✓ Increase in normal vaginal discharge
✓ Mild shortness of breath
✓ Lightheadedness or dizziness
✓ Headaches
✓ Gas, heartburn, and/or constipation
✓ Skin and hair changes

At Your Doctor Visit

Beyond the usual weigh and measure routine, your doctor will screen for gestational diabetes toward the end of this month. If she hasn't discussed counting fetal movements before, she might mention it now.

Now that you're halfway through pregnancy, you are perhaps thinking more about labor and delivery issues. It's never too early to ask your doctor questions about what's on your mind. It's also a good time to start gathering information on childbirth classes from your local hospital or birthing center. There are several different methods of childbirth education; researching them now will give you and your partner time to learn more about which one is right for you. Even if you have experience in the delivery room, you can still benefit from a refresher course. Register early, but try to pick a class date that falls in your third trimester so that the information will still be fresh in your mind once the big day arrives.

On Your Mind

There's bound to be an uncomfortable episode or two while your emotions are so close to the surface. Couple this emotional tension with your ever-growing list of things to do, and meltdown is imminent. Try to defuse the situation ahead of time by having an action plan for coping with anger-provoking situations.

Irritability

Because of all the added demands on your body, mind, and emotional equilibrium, you could be finding yourself short on patience these days. In pregnancy the proverbial molehill quickly becomes a mountain. You have absolutely no tolerance for the idiosyncrasies of others, and people you found mildly annoying before pregnancy can become absolutely impossible to be around.

If you can't stand your coworker's endless prattle about who did what to whom and got away with it, tell her you need some quiet time. And the next time your neighbor launches into her 303 easy steps for making your home look as great as hers, politely excuse yourself for a rest rather than letting your boiling point rise. Pregnancy is the perfect excuse for steering clear of people who—let's face it—are just plain annoying. During this crucial time in which your emotional and physical balance are so important, it's good to have solutions for taking care of the little things and keeping your sanity intact.

If family and friends are getting your ire up as well, it might be a sign that you are feeling overwhelmed and undersupported. Take a look at what's really getting to you. When you blow up at your partner for forgetting to stop at the dry cleaner, is it because you really have to get your winter sweaters back posthaste, or because lately you feel like you have to either nag or do it yourself to accomplish anything? If the latter, sit down and tell your partner what you're feeling, and work out some strategies for easing the burden together.

Overwhelmed

Half of your pregnancy has passed you by, the baby's room is a sea of boxes, you can't decide on a name, and your office isn't even close to being ready for your maternity leave. Step back and take stock. Are you making work—and stress—for yourself through self-imposed deadlines? Look at your to-do list in terms of small tasks rather than as an all-or-nothing duty. Prioritize what's there and dare to cross off a few things that just aren't that important right now. It's nice to have everything "just so" for baby's arrival, but your new son is only going to care about three things—being warm, well fed, and near his mom and dad.

Also remember that you aren't in this alone. If you're single, enlist family or close friends to help out. And if you are married but still aren't getting the help and support you need from your husband or family, ask for it. Although it's nice when others anticipate your needs and pitch in voluntarily, they may be wrapped up in their own preparations and anxieties about the new family addition. Don't feel guilty about reminding them that their help is needed now.

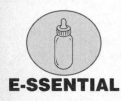

E-SSENTIAL

Having a planned C-section? You'll still benefit from prepared childbirth classes, which offer a comprehensive look at the entire birth experience, including hospital policies and procedures, newborn care, and a sneak peek at the birthing facilities. Mention your cesarean when you call for information; some programs offer special classes just for moms who are having C-sections.

Sleeping Tight

Perhaps it's nature's way of preparing you for the sleepless nights to come, but your growing belly and the pushes and prods of your little one are making it increasingly difficult to get the requisite 8 or more hours of peaceful slumber. Sleep is essential to your mental and physical fitness right now, not to mention that of your unborn child. Make your best effort to rest often and rest well.

Making Time

You work a full day at the office, go to the grocery store, go home and make dinner, stay up late working on the baby's room, and the next thing you know, it's midnight. Sleep is a priority right now, one you need to make time for. Make a regular bedtime and stick to it. Leave major cleaning, errands, and home projects for weekends or days you are off work or have extra help. If hitting the hay late is unavoidable, try to make up your sleep deficit with a weekend nap.

Getting Comfortable

The fetal sleep cycle is only between 20 and 80 minutes long, so if you aren't a sound sleeper you may find yourself awakened by baby's stretching limbs. Getting comfy can be a challenge if you were a dedicated stomach or back sleeper prepregnancy. Remember: lying on your back puts undue pressure on your inferior vena cava, the vein that shuttles blood from your lower extremities (feet and legs) to your heart, and the pressure can trigger a drop in blood pressure. It's also extremely uncomfortable for any length of time by now. Logistically and medically, the best position for sleep right now is on your side.

Hip and shoulder pain can be another source of sleepless nights, one that's difficult to avoid since you must sleep on your side. If you've tried the tips for aches and pains outlined previously and the pain is still keeping you awake, experiment with a foam cushion on your mattress for a little added padding.

You don't know what living is until you've had the luxury of stretching out full (and pregnant) on an acre of crisp, cool sheets. If you don't have one already, and the budget allows, consider upgrading to a king-size bed. The extra room will enable you to bring a body pillow or beanbag into bed to support your stomach and ease your back. Your partner will benefit, too, as he'll be less likely to wake at every toss and turn.

E-FACT

Left-side sleeping enhances blood flow exchange with the fetus. Why is the left side preferred? Because the liver resides on your right side, and sleeping on that side positions your heavy uterus right on top of it. That said, right side sleeping won't really hurt anything in a typical pregnancy, so if you wake up on your right, don't panic.

Another bedroom habit you have possibly picked up in pregnancy is that of snoring. Many women are mortified—and self-conscious—about this new development. After all, there's nothing that makes you feel more unattractive than the thunderous vibration of your own nasal passages, unless it's waking up with a trail of dried drool on your face! The snoring is related to a number of factors, including pregnancy-related nasal congestion, your increased need for oxygen, swollen airway tissues, and compression of the muscles that control breathing. Most of the miracle remedies and devices you see on TV will do little but cost you money. Your snoring will likely fade away after pregnancy. For now, invest in extra earplugs for your mate instead.

Make sure your environment is as sleep friendly as possible. The room temperature should be cool enough for your overheated metabolism; your partner might want to stock up on extra blankets to get him through occasional chilly nights. If ambient noise is a problem, get some earplugs or a white-noise conditioner to cut the clamor. Keep a night-light plugged into your room or hallway to navigate those inevitable late-night bathroom breaks with no injuries.

If you have been experiencing sleep-disturbing snoring regularly, make a point of mentioning this to your doctor. Several studies have linked chronic snoring in pregnancy to an increased risk of high blood pressure and preeclampsia. If you snored excessively prepregnancy, you could have a sleep disorder known as *sleep apnea* that should be assessed by a doctor.

More tips for preparing yourself for a good night's sleep:

✓ To avoid heartburn, don't eat immediately before bunking down, and have an extra pillow on hand to elevate your head.

✓ Make the bathroom the last stop before bed.

✓ Stock your nightstand with crackers if you still wake with an unsettled stomach.

✓ If tender breasts are keeping you awake, wear a jogging or other supportive bra to bed.

✓ Stay away from caffeine (it isn't the best thing for you right now, anyway).

✓ Don't exercise for up to 3 hours before bedtime.

Just for Dads

Although your partner is still in the relative calm and comfort of the second trimester, you may be bone tired as her tossing, turning, and expanding territorial stake of the bed have you sleeping fitfully. Some earplugs or perhaps an occasional night on the couch or guestroom bed to recoup sleep losses can be invaluable. You could also be thinking more, perhaps with some apprehension, about your impending dad duties. Instead of worrying, take action.

Practice Makes Perfect

It's often said that a new baby doesn't come with an owner's manual or instruction book, but that's not completely true. Most hospitals and birthing centers will offer you a small forest of literature on how to care for your child once you get him home. Between this, prenatal education classes, and the hundreds of baby books at your local library and bookstore, you can at least gain an understanding of how all the components are supposed to work.

If you're feeling a little insecure about your capabilities, however, getting some hands-on experience with a living, breathing baby can be a real plus. Offer to take care of a niece, nephew, or neighbor's child so that you and your partner can get some baby care practice. (Hint: don't use the word "practice" when offering babysitting services to the parents.) If you're not quite up to the flying-solo skill level yet, the next time you're visiting, take the opportunity to hold, feed, or (if you're feeling daring) change the baby.

The Second Time Around

Perhaps you're an expert at all of this dad stuff already, and you've been coasting through this pregnancy with ease. You still have some unknowns to deal with, including how your existing child or children will handle the mantle of siblinghood. Don't forget that every pregnancy is different, and what could have been smooth sailing last time may be tougher this round.

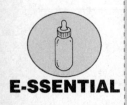

E-SSENTIAL

According to the National Sleep Foundation, up to 15 percent of women experience restless leg syndrome (RLS) in late pregnancy. Characterized by pain or unpleasant sensations in the legs, RLS may be related to nerve compression or a folate and/or iron deficiency. If RLS is keeping you awake, talk to your doctor about treatment options.

Also keep in mind that even if you don't have new-dad anxieties to contend with, your partner still has to do the heavy work. Share child care duties, take time to pamper her, and make her feel like a supermodel mom-to-be rather than the old lady who lives in a shoe.

Repeat Performance: Second or Subsequent Pregnancies

Maybe you've been around the block before and consider yourself an expert at this pregnancy stuff. You've conquered morning sickness (or at least out-lasted it) and can distinguish a Braxton-Hicks from a real contraction without running to your pregnancy books. But even if the physical side of pregnancy is familiar, the emotional and mental aspects involved with each new child are always different. Families change with each new member. Yours will be no exception.

Baby and Your Body

Women who have been through pregnancy already (*multigravida* in clinical lingo) have some definite physical benefits when it comes to carrying and delivering their babies. On average, labor is shorter, and such women are statistically less likely to have vaginal tearing and need an episiotomy.

In addition, you'll probably feel your little one stirring earlier than your first, primarily because you can identify the sensation this time. Depending on the tone of your abdominal muscles, which may be laxer after your first pregnancy, you might also start to show earlier.

Every Pregnancy Is Different . . . Or the Same

In pregnancy, practice doesn't always make perfect. Just when you think you have it down, Mother Nature can throw you a curve ball. You might have been horribly nauseated throughout your first pregnancy but not even have a gas bubble this time around. Or your second pregnancy could be filled with all sorts of strange new symptoms. Each baby has her own genetic blueprint, her own site of implantation, and her own unique placenta. The environment and life circumstances that each child is born into can be vastly different as well. It's also possible that your second pregnancy is a carbon copy of your first. So, is this pregnancy the same or different? You just have to wait and see.

VBAC or Another C-section?

"Once cesarean, always cesarean" is an out-of-date obstetric concept. Although many factors are involved in the decision to repeat a C-section (for example, a high-risk pregnancy, the fetal position, type of incision made in the first C-section, scarring of the uterus, number of previous C-sections), many women can and do try vaginal birth after cesarean (commonly known as VBAC). According to ACOG, the success rate of attempted VBAC is between 60 and 80 percent.

In the days when a classical (vertical) incision of the uterine wall was the obstetric norm, VBACs were often discouraged because of the risk of uterine rupture. Rupture might occur when a weakened scar from a previous C-section burst open under the pressure of strong contractions of the muscles of the uterus. Today the standard of care for a cesarean is a low, horizontal, midline incision across the part of the uterus where the uterine wall is thinnest. This makes rupture in VBAC highly unlikely.

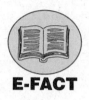

E-FACT

The rate of vaginal birth after a previous cesarean has dropped steadily since peaking in 1996, when VBAC accounted for 28.3 percent of total births. Today VBAC rates are around 8.3 percent of total births. Part of this is attributable to the overall rise in cesarean births in general: 1.4 million in 2007—one-third of all births.

Clinical studies have shown that labor-inducing agents like prostaglandins can increase the chance of uterine rupture in VBAC. For this reason, ACOG recommends avoiding their routine use in labor induction of VBAC, especially when followed by oxytocin. Misoprostol, another prostaglandin induction agent, should not be used at all in VBAC.

In women who are considered appropriate candidates for VBAC, vaginal delivery is often encouraged over C-section because of the potential complications involved with abdominal surgery (for example, infection, hemorrhage). And if you are a third-, fourth-, or more-time mom who has had a previous vaginal delivery in addition to a previous C-section, your risk of complications can actually be lower if you opt for trying labor rather than a repeat cesarean.

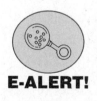

E-ALERT!

Do keep in mind that another C-section also requires a longer recovery period than in vaginal birth, something to consider when you already have children who must be cared for postpartum in addition to your new baby duties. However, recovery might seem a bit faster than after your first C-section just because you know what to expect.

If you are having a VBAC, your provider may prefer that you deliver in a hospital equipped to handle a C-section if one becomes necessary. On the other hand, for an uncomplicated pregnancy scheduled to deliver by VBAC, many midwives don't believe such a setting is necessary. Such a decision is highly dependent on your medical history and also on the laws and facility regulations in your area. If you are considered at low risk, a birthing center or even a home birth may be a reasonable choice for you. Consult your provider for her take on the situation.

VBAC isn't for everyone. At the same time, if you had a difficult labor and delivery that ended in a C-section with your first child and you really want an elective (planned) C-section this time, discuss this option with your provider. It will benefit you to explore all the pros and cons of either choice so that your decision is a fully informed one.

Sharing the News

Don't be too disappointed if your news isn't met with the fanfare that your first pregnancy announcement was greeted with. People tend to be a bit more laid back in reacting to second or subsequent pregnancies, which actually can be a better approach in helping your child or children adjust to the news.

With an Only Child

Telling your other child or children is possibly not all you imagined it would be, either. The reactions you get run the gamut from happiness to horror. But involving the kids in the pregnancy from the beginning can benefit all of you in the end. Even the child who has been begging for a little sister or brother will have some adjustments to deal with. If you know the gender of the new baby, that could also have some bearing on how your child takes the news. Children who envisioned a resident same-sex playmate can be crestfallen when their plans are detoured. Don't worry; your little one will eventually come around.

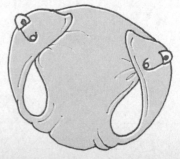

Should you reveal the new arrival's gender if you know it? You know your child and her personality best. For example, if she doesn't like surprises and takes a while to warm up to new situations, you might want to let her know so that she can prepare herself (particularly if she's making grand plans for her sister—and a brother is coming).

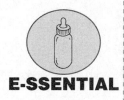

E-SSENTIAL

If you have a toddler or preschooler, think about waiting until the first trimester draws to a close to clue him in. Time passes slowly from a young child's perspective. Adding this short delay may make the wait more bearable. Of course, there is no one size that fits all. Consider your child's unique temperament in deciding when to share the news.

If you have the opportunity, exposing your child to a friend's or relative's baby may pique his curiosity about how these little people work. Children who have absolutely no interest in sharing you can be coaxed into a more optimistic attitude if you're able to involve them in the pregnancy.

With an Older Sibling

Older children can be involved with your pregnancy much earlier and will probably enjoy helping you consider new baby names, hearing the baby's heartbeat, seeing the new sibling on the ultrasound screen, and marking other milestone events of pregnancy. If they're old enough and have expressed an interest in helping out with baby care once their brother or sister arrives, you might even sign them up for a babysitting course through your local Red Cross.

In Blended Families

Blending families and stepsiblings at any age can be a challenge. Giving your children or stepchildren time to make a healthy adjustment to their new family unit prior to a pregnancy is probably the best way to set the stage for a new sibling. Even if your family is relatively young, all of you (especially stepsiblings) will likely be brought closer together by this new common bond in your family life.

Even so, along with the uncertainties that any child experiences about a new baby in the family, a stepsibling might all the more question his place in the new family unit. Will the new baby replace him in your mind? Will the baby receive the lion's share of love and attention because both her parents live in the household? Involving the kids throughout the pregnancy, stressing their importance as siblings, and being supportive when they struggle with the transition are the best ways to ensure that your family comes through pregnancy stronger than ever.

On Your Child's Mind

Getting comfortable with the idea of having a sibling, sharing parents, and potentially sharing a whole lot more will take a little time. Don't rush your child or expect instant excitement at the idea of a new baby. Each kid adjusts in her own way, on her own schedule.

Keeping your child's life relatively consistent on other fronts can help her adapt to the new baby better. Now is probably not the time to start a potty-training push, a move to a new house, or a change of day care providers. Stay on an even keel so that she doesn't get overloaded.

Of course, some transitions, such as starting school, may be unavoidable. If a change is to occur, make sure it is cast in a positive light and its significance is duly noted, even if your household is in prebaby chaos. The first day of kindergarten is a big deal and should be treated as such.

E-FACT

Some household changes, like moving your child into a big-kid bed so that the new baby can have her crib, may seem small to you but can make your child uneasy and even resentful. If she has to move into a new room before baby's arrival, give her the chance to help plan and decorate it.

Fetus Rivalry

Even before birth, your unborn child is taking a lot of your time and attention, especially in your other kids' eyes. Turning home life into a baby-centric universe in which every discussion involves their sibling's arrival is a surefire way to get your children's guards up and may even make them question their importance in the family. Of course, talking about the baby's arrival is inevitable and healthy—in moderation. Just make sure the discussions don't exclude your other children.

If pregnancy is making you experience symptoms like nausea and vomiting that have you moving slower than usual, your child may blame his sibling-to-be for your condition: "Mom can't go to the beach again. That baby is causing trouble already, and the little pipsqueak isn't even born yet!"

Assure your child that the way you are feeling is normal and is not caused by their unborn sibling directly but is just part of pregnancy. You might even relate stories of your pregnancy with him or her if it was also plagued by morning sickness or other discomforts.

What's Happening to Mom?

Young children are clueless about how a baby comes into the world. Stories of baby-dropping birds and kids popping out of cabbage patches can have them thoroughly confused. A good age-appropriate children's book on the subject can help you communicate the mechanics of the miracle of pregnancy and birth if you find yourself at a loss for words. Your local children's librarian should also be able to point you in the right direction.

When talking with your child about conception, pregnancy, and birth, there are a few issues you need to remember:

- **Be straightforward.** Don't fall back on the stork. Age makes a difference in how much your child wants or needs to know, but when you do answer questions, try to call a penis a penis, not a ding-ding, tinkler, or other adorable euphemism (as tempting as it may be). Giving your child the right words to explain what is happening to your body and his family is a way to empower him and demystify this sometimes-scary process.
- **Minimize the minutiae.** At the same time, don't take your children from Fallopian tube through baby's head crowning. Not only will they be bored, but they'll probably tune out shortly after sperm meets egg.
- **Answer all queries.** As pregnancy progresses and becomes more visible and therefore more real to your child, questions may start to form in his mind. How can the baby breathe? How will she come out? What's she doing in there? Open the door for communication and

ask your child occasionally whether she is wondering anything about your pregnancy.

- **Make it relevant.** Kids love to hear stories about their own infancy and even fetal life. Pull out the baby book and home movies and explain what life was like when they were the new arrivals.
- **Explain the emotion.** Don't forget to let your child know why you've chosen to bring another family member into the fold. Let her be aware of the intense love surrounding the choice to conceive and to bring her a sibling she can love as well.

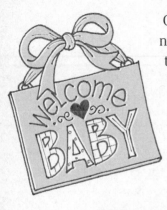

Once it becomes clear that a new baby is on the way, you could notice some behavior regressions in your younger child. Wanting to use a bottle, having potty-training accidents, and engaging in other babyish behavior is her way of saying she still needs you. Don't get angry with your child for slipping back into old habits, but do reinforce positive behaviors and point out the pluses and privileges of acting like a "big kid" (for example, "If you talk like a big kid instead of using baby talk, you can learn how to answer the telephone").

Needing Reassurance

Even the most well-adjusted, confident kid needs reassurance once in a while that she's still the apple of your eye. Don't let your world revolve around baby preparations so much that it overshadows special time spent with your other children. And make sure you give your children every opportunity to be involved with your family expansion so that they feel needed and wanted.

Involving the Sibling(s)-to-Be

Making your child a part of the pregnancy process is imperative to starting siblinghood off on a positive note. A kid who is relegated to the sidelines while everyone is focused first on your pregnancy and then on the baby is going to resent this new intruder, with good reason. Start the getting-acquainted process before birth, and let your child talk and sing to her little sibling, help decorate the new baby's digs, and take on other important tasks.

Sibling Classes

Many hospitals offer classes for new siblings as a companion to their roster of childbirth education programs. When done right, an "official" preparation —complete with nursery tour, baby (doll) practice, and in some cases a diploma—can make even the most reluctant big brother feel special and important in his imagined new sibling's eyes.

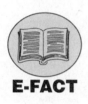

E-FACT

A good way to start the sibling relationship off on a positive note is to pick out a special gift from the new baby to her big sister, presented during their first meeting. Your new addition will be receiving copious amounts of attention, praise, and gifts, so this little gesture will symbolize a lot to your older child.

Sibling classes can also give your child a chance to air his fears among peers and receive reassurance that he isn't alone in worrying about this squalling, needy creature that's moving in soon. Discussions about how other households are handling baby preparations, sleeping arrangements, and mom's upcoming trip to the hospital can also address concerns that your child hasn't thought of or hasn't felt comfortable verbalizing.

Classes should be small enough for discussion and interaction with peers and with the instructor, and should ideally be separated into appropriate age groups.

Through the Ages

Preteens and adolescents might be more receptive to the prospect of a new sibling, simply because they're entering a phase in their development in which they are focusing less on you and more on friendships with their social circle. A fourteen- or fifteen-year-old doesn't need you the way a toddler, preschooler, or elementary school child does. You've gone from mommy to mom in her eyes, and a baby doesn't pose the same competition for your affections.

Just for the Second-Time Dad

Dads often feel that they have a bigger role to play in a second or later pregnancy as the bulk of child care falls to them while mom deals with pregnancy symptoms. This is a great opportunity for you to spend time doing things with your kids that your spouse normally gets to handle and to help them adjust to baby's upcoming arrival.

Of course, all this "together time" can have its pitfalls. While you may find yourself appreciating your wife even more when you have to take on tasks she seems to handle effortlessly on a daily basis, that awe may sour to resentment as you realize that the situation won't change back to the old way anytime soon. If you feel burdened, ignoring the problem is not the solution. Stress is bad for both of you, but particularly for the growing baby who's the focus of all these changes. Don't let any hard feelings get the better of your family.

Get help from nearby family members, or hire sitters and household help if necessary. Even a neighborhood high school student can be useful to your spouse as a mother's helper. And remember that your older kids may be ready and willing to take on new responsibilities in the family. The key is to communicate how you're feeling, without blame, and work on a way to resolve together any problem.

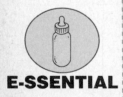

E-SSENTIAL

Don't forget that your significant other also has more to cope with this time around. It's harder to find the time for pampering when you have kids who need your attention, but get creative. Giving her a little time to herself is really essential, even if it's just for an evening walk or a 15-minute adult conversation with a close friend.

Living Large: When You Choose a Big Family

"One is wonderful, two are terrific, three—well you're starting to lose me, but I guess I see the benefits. Four? Are you NUTS?" If you have chosen to have a big family, you are probably used to this kind of reaction. Or perhaps you're just getting into the sizable stage now and haven't learned to shrug off the "When are you moving into the shoe?" comments yet.

The U.S. Census Bureau reports that in 2008 the average number of children for women nearing the end of their childbearing years was 1.9. That's well below the average of 3.1 that was reported in 1976 (the year the Census Bureau started collecting this information).

Whether your reasons are religious, rooted in your own upbringing, or simply spring from a desire to have a home bursting with life and love, the bottom line is: it's your choice and your family. Don't let others make you feel freakish or, worse yet, like you're neglecting the children you already have, just because you choose to have more than the national average. A child is one of the greatest gifts you can give your family and community.

The success of a family lies in parenting quality, not in offspring quantity (or lack of quantity). Ignore the naysayers and remember that there are pitfalls and positives to every family configuration, large and small. There are enough theories and studies on sibling personality traits and birth order psychology to fill a not-so-small library. Although they are fascinating to read, trying to base your future family structure on them is next to impossible. Not every middle child will be the easygoing mediator of the family, and not every only child will be a hopeless perfectionist. Instead, use the lessons in the books to avoid possible parenting pitfalls.

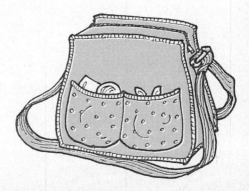

Month 6

At 6 months, you feel perhaps as though you'll be pregnant forever. And you're hitting your stride as a mom-to-be. You've embraced the practicality (if not the fashion sense) of stretchy-panel pants, have finally mastered a comfy sleep position, and have come to terms with the amazing (and somewhat disturbing) plasticity of the human body. This final trimester will come and go before you know it, so take some time this month to savor pregnancy, warts and all, and treat yourself to the indulgences that only a mother-to-be can pull off.

Baby This Month

Feeling a rhythmic lurch in your abdomen? Your little guy probably has the hiccups, a common phenomenon thought to be brought on by his drinking and/or breathing amniotic fluid. They'll go away on their own eventually; in the meantime, enjoy your little drummer boy and take advantage of the beat to let your partner feel the baby move.

The once-transparent skin of your fetus is starting to thicken, and sweat glands are developing below the skin surface. He's over a foot long now and by the end of the month will weigh up to 2 pounds.

E-FACT

Strange but true: if you're having a girl, your uterus also holds the origins of your grandchildren. By week 24 of gestation, your fetus has already developed an estimated seven million eggs in her ovaries. The eggs are enveloped in small sacs called *follicles* as pregnancy continues, and by birth the number of eggs will have decreased to around a million.

Your unborn baby might now startle (react) to a loud noise or other stimulation. Because his auditory system (the cochlea and pathways in the CNS) has developed enough to sense and even readily discriminate among sounds, he is becoming accustomed to your voice and that of others who talk to him frequently. Studies have demonstrated that newborns show a clear preference for their mothers' voices and for songs they heard while in the womb. Now is a good time to brush up on your lullaby repertoire.

Some clinical studies have found an association between exposure to excessive noise during pregnancy and high-frequency hearing loss in newborns. And while you can wear earplugs, your baby doesn't have the luxury. To stay on the safe side, it's best to avoid concerts, clubs, and other high-volume environments now. If your job involves heavy noise exposure, talk with your doctor about possible risks.

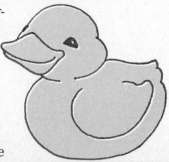

Your Body This Month

Your uterus extends well above your navel now. You may actually be seeing fetal movement across your abdomen as baby gets comfortable in his shrinking living space. As baby seems to get more nimble, you feel exceedingly klutzy—breaking everything that isn't nailed down, tripping over your own swollen feet, and upsetting low-lying knickknacks with your burgeoning belly. Blame it on your shifting center of gravity, and be careful if you're walking in slippery or icy conditions.

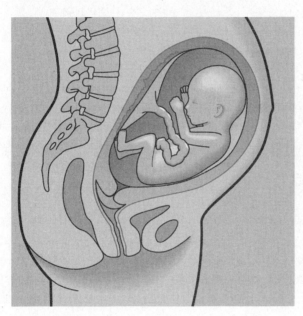

You and your baby at the 6-month mark

Your Body Changes

If the shoe fits . . . consider yourself lucky. Few women are able to fit into all their prepregnancy shoes for 9 whole months. What's behind all the swelling? The dramatic increase in blood volume you've experienced in order to nurture your child is feeding excess fluids to surrounding tissues, resulting in edema (water retention). To make matters worse, the weight of your uterus is requiring the veins in your legs to work double time to pump all that extra blood back to the heart. And, of course, another culprit is (say it together, everyone) pregnancy hormones, as estrogen increases the amount of fluid your tissues absorb.

The result of all this is puffy and sometimes aching feet. Putting your feet up when you can, wearing comfortable low-heeled shoes, and soaking your feet in cool water are all good ways to ease the discomfort. Special compression stockings, available at medical supply stores, can also be helpful.

E-ALERT!

If you experience sudden and severe swelling of the face and hands, call your doctor immediately. It may be a sign of preeclampsia (toxemia), a condition that is potentially hazardous to both you and your baby. Other signs of preeclampsia include high blood pressure, headaches, visual disturbances, and protein in the urine.

Don't restrict fluids or sodium. Although avoiding excess sodium intake is fine, you actually need slightly more sodium in your diet in pregnancy to maintain your electrolyte balance. Fluids are crucial as well, to prevent dehydration and keep you and baby well.

What You Feel Like

You might have added leg cramps to your laundry list of pregnancy complaints. Stretching out your calf muscles can often quash a cramp, so the next time one hits, extend your legs and point your toes toward your head. Some providers suggest calcium supplements to ease cramping, but clinical studies are inconclusive as to whether this treatment is effective (although it can't hurt, given your increased calcium needs right now). A number of studies have found, however, that oral magnesium supplementation can be useful in alleviating cramps in some women. Check with your health care provider to see what she suggests.

Leg cramps can also be triggered by compression of your sciatic nerve—a condition commonly known as *sciatica*. Sciatica can also cause numbness and burning pain down the length of your leg and in your lower back and buttocks. Try stretching, a warm compress, or a tub soak for relief. If sciatica becomes more than a minor annoyance, talk to your health care provider. A date with a physical therapist may be in order.

If your leg pain is accompanied by swelling, redness, and skin that is warm to the touch, call your health care provider to report your symptoms.

You could be experiencing deep vein thrombosis (DVT), a blood clot in your leg that impedes circulation and has the potential to embolize (break off and block a major blood vessel). Pregnant women are five times more likely to develop DVT than their nonpregnant peers due to a slowdown of blood flow and an increase in clotting factors. However, DVT itself is relatively rare, occurring in less than one of every 1,000 pregnancies. If DVT is diagnosed, intravenous anticoagulant drugs are typically prescribed to treat the clot, and bed rest is advised.

E-QUESTION

Can the seat belt in my car hurt the baby?
Definitely continue to buckle up for safety throughout your pregnancy. The lap belt should fit snugly under your belly bulge, and the shoulder belt should be positioned between your breasts. Don't worry about the belt hurting the baby; the uterus and fluid-filled amniotic sac are excellent shock absorbers.

Other symptoms on the menu yet again this month include:

✓ Nausea
✓ Fatigue
✓ Frequent urination
✓ Tender and/or swollen breasts
✓ Bleeding gums
✓ Excess mucus and saliva
✓ Increase in normal vaginal discharge
✓ Mild shortness of breath
✓ Lightheadedness or dizziness
✓ Headaches
✓ Forgetfulness
✓ Gas, heartburn, and/or constipation
✓ Skin and hair changes
✓ Round ligament pain or soreness
✓ Lower-back aches
✓ Mild swelling of legs, feet, and hands

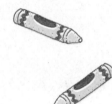

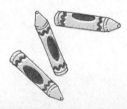

At Your Doctor Visit

There is more of the same this month as your provider checks your weight and fundal height, listens to baby's heartbeat, and finds out about any new pregnancy symptoms you are experiencing. If you're reporting swelling, your provider may check your feet and hands. And, of course, no prenatal visit is complete without a urine sample and blood pressure check. If you weren't given a glucose challenge test to screen for gestational diabetes last month, it will probably be administered now.

On Your Mind

Now that your belly is too big to not notice, it becomes a conversation piece. At first you may be surprised to find women you don't know asking about your due date or the gender of your baby. The next question will inevitably be "Is this your first?" Welcome to the sisterhood of motherhood.

Take advantage of all the attention. As you get closer to your baby's birthday, you could find your questions (and possibly your anxieties) about labor and delivery multiplying. Other moms are usually more than willing to share the unvarnished truth, so when someone engages you in conversation about your pregnancy, ask questions back. Just keep in mind that every birth is different, so your experience will be unique.

The "What If" Game

Every new-mom-to-be spends some time worrying about the health of her unborn child, especially if she's in a high-risk pregnancy. Take comfort in the facts that you've almost made it to the third trimester and your chances of delivering a healthy and happy baby are increasing each and every day. Obsessing over what could go wrong rather than focusing on living well will accomplish nothing but add stress, insomnia, and anxiety—three things that are bad for you and baby. Read on for some stress-busting techniques to release your worries and relieve your mind.

Enjoying Your Pregnancy

As you sidle up to the third trimester starting line, try to take advantage of these final days of relative comfort and sit back and savor—yes, savor—your pregnancy.

Pamper Yourself

Splurge for a day spa treatment. Spend a lazy afternoon curled up with a good book. Cool off with a dish of your favorite Ben & Jerry's flavor while you enjoy a nice relaxing soak in the tub. Take a scenic weekend drive with no deadlines or particular destination. Pampering yourself can relieve pregnancy symptoms, give you (alone or with your partner) special time to reflect on your future, and recharge you for what lies ahead.

Make sure you treat yourself to the little conveniences right now, too. Use the valet service to park instead of hiking from the lot, or shop at stores with expectant mother parking front and center. Too tired to cook at the end of the day? Order healthy carryout fare from your favorite restaurant. If it's only lunchtime and you're already beat, arrange for an away-from-home playdate for the kids for a few hours and have a midafternoon snooze. It might feel decadent at first, but taking the easy way out is a good thing right now.

Don't Stress

It bears repeating—again—that getting stressed out these days just isn't worth it for you or your growing child. Of course, pampering yourself is one good way to lighten the load. But some women find they just can't enjoy a good old-fashioned self-indulgence day because they're too busy worrying about all the things they should be doing instead. If you fall into this category, don't add to your burden through forced relaxation that will only leave you tense and perhaps out several hundred dollars, to boot.

Instead, use that money to whittle down your to-do list. Hire a cleaning service, send out the laundry, pay someone to do that painting in the baby's room, have the groceries delivered instead of schlepping to the supermarket. If your financial resources are limited, let your loved ones know you could really use their help right now, and don't be shy about delegating tasks when assistance is offered.

Spending Time with Siblings-to-Be

Watching your child marvel at the changes in your body while he considers the possibilities of a new little sister or brother can be one of the most fun and fulfilling parts of pregnancy. Yet even the most enthusiastic sibling-to-be has some doubts about how he will fit into the new family unit. Unfortunately, those insecurities may only be intensified as you spend more time in the coming months visiting the doctor, going to childbirth classes, and tying down loose ends before the big day. Make sure you and your child (or children) have an opportunity each day to play, read, or just talk. You'll each benefit from this special time together.

Couple Time

With you in the pregnancy limelight and all the attention that your agile, rib-thumping fetus demands, perhaps you have inadvertently started to think of you and the baby as a couple. Your husband or partner is not an orbiting moon, although he may feel like one from time to time. Make sure he knows that he plays an essential role in this pregnancy, and take the time to reconnect with him emotionally and physically.

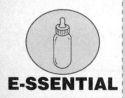

E-SSENTIAL

If these are your final few months as a childless couple, take advantage of your freedom and spend some time doing your favorite grown-up things, activities that don't involve visiting the doctor's office or shopping for cribs and strollers.

If you're both still ready, willing, and up to the challenge, sex can be more fun than ever. You don't have to worry about birth control, and the creativity required to find a comfortable position can inspire you to new heights. If the two of you are so inclined, oral sex is a good option; just make sure your partner is aware that he should not blow into your vagina due to the rare but real risk of an air embolism. Women in high-risk pregnancies should consult their doctor about the safety of intercourse right now.

Just for Dads

Pregnancy is a one-of-a-kind time in your life as well as in your partner's. This long, strange trip—from "My boys can swim!" to "Breathe, honey, breathe!"—brings elation, anxiety, anticipation, and much more.

It also gives you the opportunity to see your partner in a whole new light: to watch her grow physically and personally as she makes the amazing transformation to motherhood. Her strength and sheer stamina in this 9-month marathon can have you feeling both proud and protective.

A Brand New Lifestyle

Yes, life will change significantly once your child arrives. No running out to catch a late movie and dinner at your favorite Mexican spot. You've got Disney matinees and Happy Meals on your dance card. But the first time your daughter smiles at you, says "daddy," or laughs out loud at jokes that no one else would, it will all be so very worth it. And before you know it, you'll actually start to enjoy this second edition of your childhood, from the parenting perspective.

Dads Should Enjoy Pregnancy, Too

Unfortunately, even though the waiting room–pacing dads of the 1950s are now history, fathers often get shut out of the pregnancy experience. The result can be frustration and anxiety. Many fathers-to-be experience significant stress related to the upcoming pressures of parenthood, but everyone's focus on mom and baby can minimize your concerns and leave you feeling excluded.

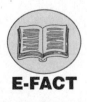

E-FACT

Planning on taking her out for a nice romantic dinner? Pick a restaurant that is completely smoke-free, and make reservations so that she won't be waiting on her feet for too long. Be sure to request a booth to give her more room to spread out. With her sometimes-fickle stomach, now is probably not the time to get adventurous with new cuisines.

It isn't just a matter of the "What about me?" syndrome. Dads who do try to connect with the pregnancy on a deeper level are sometimes ridiculed for their efforts. Ever get laughed at when you tell others that "we're pregnant"? Or perhaps you're the type who snickers when the other guy announces his pregnancy (come on, you know who you are). Either way, you might end up internalizing your questions and fears due to a misguided sense of stoicism, consequently distancing yourself from the pregnancy experience.

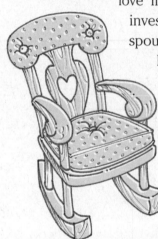

Obviously, you'll never be able to fully experience pregnancy in a physical sense (nor will you probably want to, after watching the woman you love live through it), but you can increase your emotional investment in this pregnancy by communicating with your spouse or partner about your hopes, dreams, and anxieties. Feeling stressed about your ability to parent, about how your relationship with your partner can change, or about possible financial changes affecting your family is completely normal. Talking about these issues as a couple can bring you closer together and help alleviate your worries.

Multiple Choice:
Two, Three, Four, or More

News of impending twins, triplets, and other multiples is certainly a thrilling and momentous surprise for any couple. Disbelief, pride, and panic are just a few of the feelings you might experience on the road to parenting multiples—not to mention the physical ramifications of having more than one baby on board. Your pregnancy may in fact mean more frequent visits to the doctor and a higher-maintenance prenatal routine, but the joys of being a multiples' mom make it all worthwhile.

Splitting Eggs and Sharing Sacs

Multiples are either monozygotic (formed from a single egg and sperm) or dizygotic (formed from two separate eggs and two sperm). Monozygotic multiples, more commonly known as *identicals*, can be further classified by the way they share their common space and maternal resources.

Identical Twins

Identical (monozygotic) twins form when a single fertilized egg (zygote) splits in two. Because they are cut from the same piece of genetic fabric, they are always the same gender. Monozygotic twins also share a placenta. Depending on when the zygote splits, they may share an amniotic sac and/or the chorionic membrane (monoamniotic/monochorionic), or they may each have their own personal space and membranes (diamniotic/dichorionic). Twins who split more than a week after fertilization will probably share both the amnion and the chorion, while twins who split early on are more likely to have separate quarters.

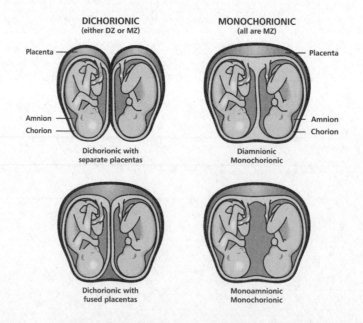

Monozygotic, or identical, twins may each have their own set of fetal membranes, or they may share an amniotic sac (monoamniotic), a chorion membrane (monochorionic), or both.

A single zygote that produces twins usually splits within days of fertilization but may wait up to 2 weeks. Zygotes that split beyond 14 days increase the risk of resulting in conjoined twins, or twins who haven't separated completely and develop with shared body parts or organ systems. Fraternal twins, because they start life as two eggs fertilized by two sperm, do not run the risk of conjoinment.

Fraternal Multiples

Fraternal (dizygotic) twins are basically siblings in the womb. Each one is created from a separate egg fertilized with its own sperm. Fraternal twins are three times more common than identical twins. They have their own placentas, can be the same or different genders, and may not look any more alike than siblings born individually.

Who Has Multiples?

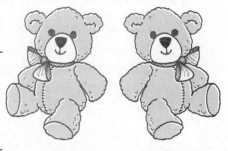

Your chances of "twinning" are actually not bad; about one in ninety births results in twins. If fraternal twins run in your family, your odds are slightly higher. The number of twins and births of multiples has skyrocketed over the past several decades, and the incidence of higher-order multiples—triplets, quadruplets, or more—grew more than 400 percent between 1980 and 1998 but has stabilized since 1999. Twins are more common than ever, however, with 138,660 twin births occurring in 2008.

Why the bonus baby boom? The CDC attributes approximately two-thirds of all higher-order multiples in the United States to the use of fertility treatments, also known as *assisted reproductive technology* (ART). Nearly 32 percent of all successful pregnancies from ART result in a multiple fraternal birth.

National statistics also reveal that more women are waiting until their thirties and forties to have children, and the increasing twin rate perhaps reflects that reality. Women over age 35, especially those who had a previous multiples' birth, have an increased chance of having multiples.

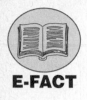

Several studies comparing birth outcomes in triplet pregnancies have found that moms over age forty have more favorable fetal growth parameters and better birth-weight outcomes than younger triplet moms.

Although birth outcomes in a singleton pregnancy involve more risk as maternal age increases, studies indicate that the opposite seems to hold true for pregnancies of multiples among older moms. This could be due in part to the increased use of ART in older women, and the fact that ART multiples rarely share the same amniotic sac—a risk factor for a number of prenatal complications in multiples' pregnancies.

Your Body in a Multiples' Pregnancy

You are living larger than you ever imagined. With all those arms and legs flailing about, you feel as if you're housing a team of tiny Olympic hopefuls. Although it may not feel like it when your crowd is going wild and your back is killing you, a multiples' pregnancy is a unique gift. That your body can accommodate and nurture not just one, but two, three, or possibly more human beings is nothing short of miraculous.

Moms-to-be of multiples experience the same pregnancy symptoms as women with only one fetus, but these can be more intense and occur earlier in the pregnancy. Excessive nausea and vomiting, in particular, are often early signs that your unborn child has company. However, many women with singleton pregnancies can experience severe morning sickness as

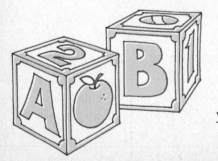

well. More significant markers of multiples' pregnancies would include the presence of more than one fetal heart tone during a prenatal examination and measuring too large for your suspected gestational age after week 24. High levels of alpha-fetoprotein on an AFP, triple-screen, or quad screen blood test can also be an indication that you have some stowaways.

Doctor Visits

If you've been diagnosed with a multiples' pregnancy, you'll be visiting your doctor more frequently. Although your appointment schedule will depend on your specific medical history and the risk factors involved in your pregnancy, you might be making the visit twice monthly in early pregnancy (as opposed to just a monthly visit for the first trimester with singleton pregnancies). Then you will shift to weekly visits early in the third trimester.

Diagnosis

While a number of symptoms and screening tests point to a multiples' pregnancy, a definitive diagnosis is usually made by ultrasound. During the ultrasound procedure, the technician will try to determine whether or not the fetuses are sharing a single amniotic sac, putting them at higher risk for some complications.

Do You Need a Perinatologist?

A perinatologist—an ob-gyn who specializes in high-risk pregnancies—is a good choice for many women expecting multiples. If your medical history is complicated or if you are expecting triplets or more, the expertise of a perinatologist can be quite valuable. When choosing a perinatologist, it should also be someone with whom you feel comfortable and able to communicate. There may be a specialist in the practice that your original doctor or midwife belongs to; this can make the transition easier.

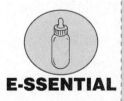

E-SSENTIAL

Moms of multiples can be a great source of information, support, and advice for the unique issues that you face, both during pregnancy and after birth. You don't have to stake out the local parks looking for twins; a local or regional "parents of multiples club" can put you in touch with someone in your area.

If you decide against a specialist, talk with your provider about his experience delivering multiples, his cesarean rate for this type of birth, and his planned course of action for your specific case. In some cases your provider might feel that your medical history warrants a referral to a perinatologist who has a high level of expertise to handle your pregnancy and delivery, but he may be willing to continue seeing you for prenatal care in conjunction with your specialist.

Problems in Multiples' Pregnancies

Multiples' pregnancies have a shorter gestation time than singleton pregnancies, simply because mom hasn't enough room and resources to house the brood for 40 weeks. On average, twin pregnancies are usually delivered at week 38, triplets at week 35, and quadruplets at week 34. The biggest risks by far in a multiples' pregnancy are preterm labor and premature birth. Gestational diabetes and preeclampsia are also risks.

Problems Mom May Face

If your body is nourishing two or more children, you need to treat it with a little extra TLC. Take an additional 600 calories daily of healthy foods (beyond average prepregnancy calorie intake), and drink plenty of water. The latter is particularly important because dehydration can trigger preterm contractions.

Moms-to-be of multiples are at greater risk for developing anemia and should speak to their provider about iron supplementation to ensure that their needs are covered. Increasing your intake of iron-rich foods is a good way to ward off anemia. Try rotating iron-rich foods such as baked beans, blackstrap molasses, wheat germ, raisins, beef, and leafy green veggies (like spinach, kale, and broccoli) into your diet.

The cervix has heavy work to do in a multiples' pregnancy. Having twins puts you at increased risk of preterm labor. Some physicians have recommended a series of screenings of the cervical length using transvaginal ultrasound to try to detect early cases of preterm labor. A screening of the cervical length at around week 20 appears to be predictive of who will deliver preterm. In women with a short cervix (approximately 25 millimeters or less at week 24), some reinforcements may be required. If cervical shortening is suspected, a transvaginal ultrasound, in which the Doppler wand is inserted into the vagina rather than moved across the belly, is used to assess cervical length and monitor the progress of the cervix. Cerclage, a procedure involving suturing (stitching) the cervix closed to avoid preterm dilation, is not routinely indicated for multiples' pregnancy but is sometimes performed for preterm cervical shortening and dilation.

E-SSENTIAL

Although due dates are typically based on a 10-lunar-month calendar, most people consider pregnancy a 9-month, three-trimester affair. That's why you'll find your pregnancy divided into 9 calendar months in this book.

Cerclage is usually performed in the second trimester. It appears that the earlier that cerclage is performed in the pregnancy, the more potential it has for success. Studies are inconclusive as to whether *rescue* cervical cerclage (an emergency procedure performed after the cervix has dilated prematurely) is effective in improving birth outcomes.

Almost half of all multiples' pregnancies result in preterm labor (before week 37). If you start having contractions or other signs of preterm labor, your provider might try to halt labor until you're further along in your pregnancy by one or more of the following methods:

- **Bed rest:** Strict bed rest may be imposed to keep the pressure off your cervix. This could be at home (with a few bathroom passes granted) or in a hospital. A fetal monitor may be used to keep an eye on the team's progress. Your provider may also recommend that you keep your feet elevated while in bed.
- **Fluids:** You may be hooked up to an intravenous line and/or fed fluids to keep you hydrated.
- **Tocolytic medication:** Tocolytic drugs like magnesium sulfate ($MgSO_4$), indomethacin, and nifedipine may be administered by mouth or intravenously to stop contractions.

- **Antibiotics:** If your membranes have ruptured prematurely (preterm premature rupture of membranes, PPROM, occurs when the amniotic sac breaks before labor begins and more than 3 weeks before your due date), antibiotics can help ward off infection and prolong the latent phase of labor. They are also used to prevent group B strep infection in the preterm newborn.

An amniocentesis can determine whether the fetal lungs are developed enough to breathe in the outside world. If results indicate that the lungs are still immature, injections of corticosteroids may be administered to accelerate surfactant production while labor is held off as long as possible. ACOG recommends steroid treatment for women expected to deliver between weeks 24 and 34.

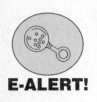

E-ALERT!

There are some situations in which tocolysis should not be attempted, even if you are considerably preterm. If monitoring indicates that your fetus is in distress, if you have signs of infection of the amniotic fluid, or if you are bleeding excessively, tocolyctic drugs are not recommended. In most of these cases, immediate delivery is required.

In amniocentesis of multiples, a blue dye is injected into each amniotic sac after a fluid sample is withdrawn. If the same sac is accidentally tested twice, the appearance of the dye will tip off the physician to the error. It's important that all sacs be tested whenever practical, as multiples often develop at different rates and may have achieved various levels of fetal lung maturity.

Problems Babies May Face

Up to 70 percent of monoamniotic twins and higher-order multiples experience umbilical cord knotting, twisting, or entanglement. In severe cases, kinks or tangles in the cord can cut off blood supply to one or both fetuses. Ultrasound can determine the presence or absence of a dividing membrane (amniotic sac) between multiples. If a multiples' monoamniotic pregnancy is detected, it will be followed closely with routine ultrasounds to check for umbilical cord complications. Regular nonstress testing (NST) may also be employed to evaluate fetal health.

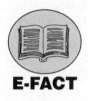

The length of expected gestation decreases with each additional fetus carried in a pregnancy. According to the March of Dimes, nearly 60 percent of twins, over 90 percent of triplets, and virtually all quadruplets and higher multiples are born preterm (before week 37 of gestation).

Twin-to-twin transfusion syndrome (TTTS) is a rare condition affecting approximately 10 percent of those identical twins who share a chorionic membrane and placenta. In TTTS an abnormality in the placenta causes irregularities in fetal blood circulation, and blood is shunted between the fetuses through placental vessels that connect them. The result is that one fetus experiences cardiovascular overload and potential heart failure, while the other receives insufficient blood flow. TTTS is not limited to twins and can occur in higher-order multiples' pregnancies as well.

In addition to its involvement with TTTS, the placenta's position and construction can impact the growth of one or more multiples. Maternal blood flow and nutrition may be unequally distributed among fetuses, resulting in an uneven growth rate among them. Multiples can also be at a higher risk for intrauterine growth retardation (IUGR).

Vanishing twin syndrome may ensue from the death of one twin that was previously viable. When it occurs early in pregnancy, the body is typically reabsorbed into the uterine wall. Some minor bleeding and cramping may signal the process. More serious complications can result if vanishing twin syndrome happens later in pregnancy, including cerebral palsy in the surviving twin and potential circulatory problems in the mother.

Other conditions that multiples are considered at high risk for include congenital abnormalities and placental problems (for example, placenta previa, placental abruption).

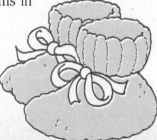

Delivering Multiples

Nothing is routine in a multiples' pregnancy, and the surprises will likely keep coming through labor and delivery as well. Close communication with both your health care provider and a neonatologist (a physician who specializes in newborn and preemie care) about the possible scenarios that you and your children face at birth will leave you better equipped to make informed decisions.

Cesarean Versus Vaginal Delivery

About half of all twins are born via cesarean section, and the number goes up considerably for triplets or more. Because of the risk of umbilical cord entanglement, multiples that share an amniotic sac are usually delivered by C-section at or before week 34.

Whether other multiples are delivered vaginally will depend on how they are positioned in the womb. If the first baby is breech (feet or buttocks first), your provider will probably prefer a C-section. If at least the first baby is vertex (head down), a vaginal delivery may be performed. Women who feel strongly about having a vaginal delivery of their multiples should speak with their provider early on in the pregnancy about the issue.

A quick ultrasound in the labor and delivery room will reveal your babies' positions. In some cases when the first baby is born but the second is breech, external cephalic version (turning the fetus by pressing on the surface of your abdomen) may be attempted to turn a stubborn twin. The fetal heart rate in the second twin will be monitored during the procedure.

Premature Birth

Babies who are born prematurely are at risk for respiratory distress syndrome (RDS) due to lung immaturity. Treatment for RDS takes several forms, depending on the severity of the condition. Animal-derived or synthetic surfactants may be administered shortly after birth to hasten lung maturation. An oxygen tube that fits under and into the nostrils can provide continuous positive airway pressure (CPAP) to force open the alveoli (air sacs) of the lungs. A newborn might also require intubation and breathing assistance with a mechanical respirator until lung function can develop further.

Preemies who develop RDS are also at risk for a lung disease called *bronchopulmonary dysplasia* (BPD). BPD occurs in up to 30 percent of infants who survive RDS and is triggered by trauma to the immature lungs from infection, respiratory therapy, or the stress of oxygen itself. Symptoms include wheezing, rapid breathing, cough, and straining of abdominal and neck muscles.

Postpartum Hemorrhage

Women who have delivered multiples are at an increased risk for postpartum hemorrhage (excessive bleeding) after delivery. Some of the tocolytic medications (for example, magnesium sulfate) can increase the risk of bleeding by inhibiting uterine muscle function. Once the placenta is delivered, the uterus must continue to contract in order to tamp down and seal off placental blood vessels. In a womb that is overstretched from multiples, the myometrium—the smooth muscle layer responsible for contractions—may not function efficiently. Postpartum hemorrhage can be the result.

If postpartum hemorrhage does occur, the uterus will be double-checked for any remaining pieces of the placenta (another cause of postpartum bleeding) and massaged to control the bleeding. Oxytocin or prostaglandin may also be administered to stimulate contractions.

When Babies Are in the NICU

You've waited and waited to hold your babies in your arms, and now they're in the neonatal intensive care unit (NICU), behind glass and bound up by wires and tubes. Be assured that even though they may be dependent on machines, your presence and parental touch are critical in speeding their recovery and eventual discharge.

"Kangaroo care," skin-to-skin parental-to-preemie contact, has been shown to have a positive impact on parent-child bonding and to improve the motor and cognitive development of premature babies. But early on, some very premature babies may not yet be ready for the sensory overload of touching. Be assured that they will want and need it as time goes on, and NICU staff and neonatal physical therapists can instruct you on nurturing forms of touch with your babies.

Never forget that your presence is essential to making this scary, sterile world a loving, temporary home for your babies. Holding their tiny hands, getting involved with their care and feeding, and learning how to care for any unique medical needs are all critical tasks right now. The skilled nursing staff of the NICU can be a tremendous resource as you become comfortable with your babies' care. Tap their expertise while you have the opportunity.

Barring any other serious medical problems, your new family members will be discharged from the hospital once they've reached a predetermined weight goal (usually around 2,000 grams, or 4.4 pounds) and are able to maintain their body temperature, to feed, and to breathe well on their own. If any of your children require special medical monitoring or attention after discharge, home visits from a nurse can help you become adjusted to their care routines.

Surviving the First Month Home

Be it hired help, grandparents, or friends, you absolutely must have backup support when you're bringing home multiples. Ideally you'll organize your recruits well before birth, but this isn't always possible given the unpredictability of due dates with multiples. Think about designating a trusted friend or relative to delegate tasks—someone who's organized and dependable. Try not to stick your spouse with the job; both of you will have your hands full when the kids are finally here.

Schedules, Schedules, Schedules

Depending on the number of babies you're juggling and whether you're breastfeeding or bottle-feeding, it might seem easier at first to just feed them all on demand. However, that strategy can eventually be at the expense of sleep and sanity. Without a little nudging, they will continue to follow their own timetable, the one that has you grabbing your shuteye in 20-minute stretches.

So, how do you get your little ones with the program? A rigid feeding and sleep schedule is doomed to failure; newborns need to know you're there for them no matter what the agenda says. A more practical and flexible approach is to wake up all the babies once one awakens to eat. Feeding them all simultaneously and then laying them back down to sleep will get them on track toward a feeding schedule that's more or less in sync.

Breast, Bottle, or Both?

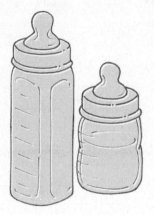

The moment you learn of multiples, breast-feeding takes on a whole new dimension. Visions of becoming a 24-hour, all-you-can-eat buffet for this litter of babies can have you revisiting your plans to nurse exclusively. Before you make any rash decisions, know that mothers of multiples can and do breastfeed (and live to tell about it!).

At the same time, don't let anyone tell you that it will be easy. It will take a lot of hard work and persistence—and an equal amount of support from family and friends—to nurse your babies successfully. But the health, bonding, and cost benefits can make breastfeeding multiples well worth your while.

Why breastfeed your brood? First of all, breastmilk is cheaper and more convenient for a single baby; multiply that time and money savings by two or more, and you end up with quite a deal. In addition, multiples can get an even bigger immunity boost from breastmilk because of their tendency to be preterm and low-birth-weight babies, two factors that raise their risk for other health problems. And breastfeeding provides special one-on-one time with each child, a rare event in multiples' land.

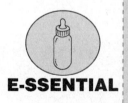

E-SSENTIAL

Your babies will probably not sleep longer than 2 hours at a stretch to start, so having them in your bedroom or getting a comfortable bed-roll or inflatable mattress for the nursery floor is a good idea for those nights when even finding your way back to bed seems too time intensive.

Many moms of twins find that nursing both children at once (tandem nursing) is the most efficient way of taking care of feeding time. This can be a little tricky to master at the outset, but you'll get better with practice. An appointment with a lactation consultant is also a good idea for breastfeeding mothers of multiples to get pointers on scheduling, logistics, and more.

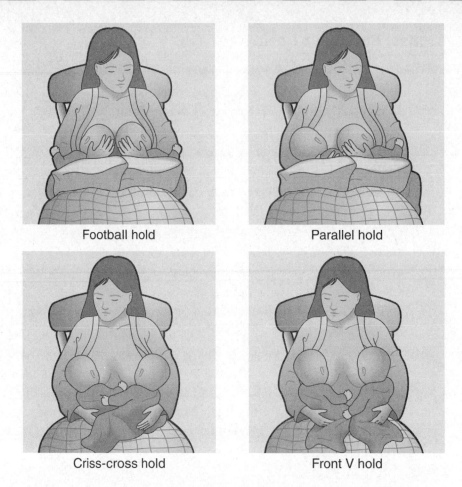

Football hold

Parallel hold

Criss-cross hold

Front V hold

Mothers of multiples can nurse two babies simultaneously in a number of positions – including the football, parallel, criss-cross, and front V holds.

Bottle-feeding can have its advantages as well, particularly with higher-order multiples. The biggest benefit is that your husband or other helpers can get in on the action, a huge plus if you're trying to get two or more babies on the same feeding and sleeping schedule. And if you have an impatient eater in your crew, you don't have to worry about making him wait his turn while the others nurse.

Really want to provide your children with the health benefits of breast-milk, but find the physical toll of nursing multiples overwhelming? Some women choose to rotate a formula feeding among their multiples while the others feed at the breast. However, this can result in a diminished milk supply over time. Consider augmenting a few breastfeedings a day with a bottle filled with pumped milk instead.

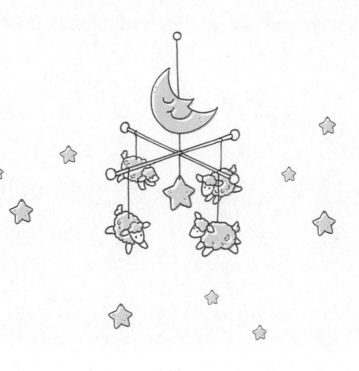

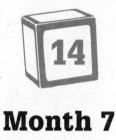

Month 7

It's the homestretch, the final act, the big countdown —the third trimester. You've made a lot of decisions so far, and there are even more to be made this month. Full speed ahead with labor-and-delivery preparations as you sort through your options for childbirth classes and start to assemble a birth plan. You may feel some Braxton-Hicks contractions as your body starts prepping for the hard work of labor. Consider them a dress rehearsal for the big event.

Baby This Month

Weighing in at 4 pounds and measuring about 16 inches long, your baby is growing amazingly fast now. Her red, wrinkled skin is losing its fine lanugo covering as more insulating fat accumulates. And her eyelids, closed for so long, can now open and afford her a dim view of the place she will call home for just a few more months.

Dramatic developments in the brain and central nervous system are also occurring, as baby's nerve cells are sheathed with a substance called *myelin* that speeds nerve impulses. A 7-month-old fetus feels pain, can cry, and responds to stimulation from light or sound outside the womb.

Her gymnastics may subside as her space gets smaller, but you're feeling her more intensely now; her movements might even be visible to both you and your partner. Periodically tiny elbows and feet will turn your belly into an interactive relief map. Gently pushing back can provide endless entertainment for all three of you.

Even though your fetus is producing lung surfactant, a liquid mixture of lipids and proteins that coats the lungs and makes it easier to breathe, and developing alveoli (air sacs), her lungs still aren't developed enough to breathe in the outside world. If complications require an early delivery now, steroids might be administered intravenously to boost surfactant production. Chemical surfactants can also be used after birth.

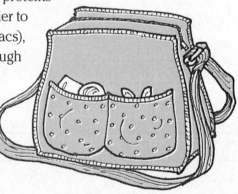

Your Body This Month

You're likely feeling perpetually stuffed and slightly out of breath as your uterus relocates all your internal organs. The relief and energy felt in the second trimester can start to fade now. Just remember, you're almost there!

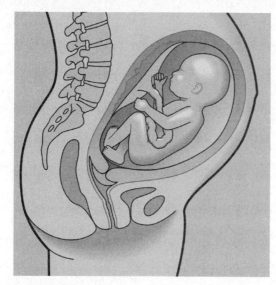

You and your baby
as you kick off the
third trimester

Your Body Changes

The top of the fundus is halfway between your bellybutton and your breast-bone, displacing your stomach, intestines, and diaphragm. Your expanding abdomen has formed a shelf, handy for resting your arms on and balancing a cold beverage at the movies. On the down side, you'll be catching a lot of crumbs, and your napkin just doesn't seem to stay on your lap anymore.

Not only are your breasts heavier, but also they are more glandular and getting ready to feed your baby. In this last trimester your nipples may begin to leak colostrum, the yellowish, nutrient-rich fluid that precedes real breast-milk. You may find the leaking more apparent when you're sexually aroused. To reduce backaches and breast tenderness, make sure you wear a well-fitting bra (even to bed, if it helps). If you are planning on breastfeeding, you might want to consider buying some supportive nursing bras now that can take you through the rest of pregnancy and right into the postpartum period.

E-FACT

If you're picking up some nursing bras, be sure to test-drive the clasps for easy nursing access. Try to unfasten and slip the nursing flaps down with one hand. This may seem unimportant now, but when you're in a crowded shopping mall juggling packages and trying to discreetly put baby to breast single-handedly, you'll be thankful you had the foresight.

What You Feel Like

Your body is warming up for labor, and you may start to experience Braxton-Hicks contractions. These painless and irregular contractions feel as if your uterus is making a fist and then gradually relaxing. If your little one is fairly active, you might think that she is stretching herself sideways at first. A quick check of your belly will reveal a visible tightening.

Braxton-Hicks can begin as early as week 20 and continue right up until your due date, although these contractions are more commonly felt in the final month of pregnancy. Some first-time moms-to-be are afraid they won't be able to tell the difference between Braxton-Hicks and actual labor contractions. As any woman who has been through labor can attest, when the real thing comes, you'll know it. Rule of thumb: if it hurts, it's labor.

Starting at week 20, the uterus has a basic rhythm. The smooth muscle of the uterus is similar to your intestinal tract in that both involuntarily contract in a wavelike pattern designed to facilitate movement of what's inside (be it breakfast or your baby). These early rhythmic and generally painless contractions are called Braxton-Hicks when they do not cause any changes to the cervix and are occurring at irregular intervals. They can even be uncomfortable at times but will usually subside if you change positions, another way to distinguish Braxton-Hicks from the real thing. The actual definition of labor, even when it is premature, is the onset of regular, painful, uterine contractions that lead to a change in the cervix.

If your contractions suddenly seem to be coming at regular intervals and they start to cause you pain or discomfort, they could be the real thing. Lie down on your left side for about a half hour with a clock or watch on hand, and time the contractions from the beginning of one to the beginning of the next. If the interludes are more or less regular, call your health care provider. And if contractions of any type are accompanied by blood or amniotic fluid leakage, contact your practitioner immediately.

The list is growing. Other symptoms that may continue this month include:

✓ Fatigue
✓ Frequent urination
✓ Tender and/or swollen breasts
✓ Bleeding gums

✓ Excess mucus and saliva
✓ Increase in normal vaginal discharge
✓ Mild shortness of breath
✓ Lightheadedness or dizziness
✓ Headaches
✓ Forgetfulness
✓ Gas, heartburn, and/or constipation
✓ Skin and hair changes
✓ Round ligament pain or soreness
✓ Lower-back aches
✓ Mild swelling of legs, feet, and hands
✓ Leg cramps

At Your Doctor Visit

Starting with this initial third-trimester visit, your trips to the doctor might start to step up to twice monthly. Your provider will probably want to know whether you've been experiencing any Braxton-Hicks contractions, and he will cover the warning signs of preterm labor and what you should do if you experience them. If you're unsure about what type of childbirth class you'd like to take, you might want to bring your questions to your provider for his take. Just remember, the decision is ultimately up to you and your partner.

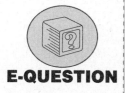

E-QUESTION

Why are people always touching me, and how can I get them to stop?
People are fascinated with the life force of pregnancy, and you're radiating it, big time. Most people will ask permission before touching, but to stop the belly rubbers who strike without warning, take a step back or turn away. Hopefully, they'll get the hint.

Women who are Rh-negative will need treatment this month with Rh immune globulin (RhIg; RhoGAM). An injection is typically given at about week 28 to protect the fetus from developing hemolytic disease—a condition in which the mother's antibodies attack the fetal red blood cells.

On Your Mind

This month will bring new questions and uncertainties as you ponder your ideal birth experience. Are you looking forward to a completely chemical-free birth, or are you already exploring your painkilling options? Is your provider open to your needs and willing to make reasonable accommodations to meet them? Do you want only your partner in attendance, or would you like additional support? Whatever your idea of perfect labor and delivery is, make sure the direction of your birth plan is driven by the needs of your partner and you and not by the expectations of others.

E-ALERT!

Don't miss the boat on insurance. Many childbirth classes, sibling classes, and breastfeeding classes are completely covered by your health insurance provider. If cost is holding you back, check out your coverage. Even if you aren't covered, courses are usually relatively inexpensive, and many facilities offer sliding-fee scales for those who qualify.

Keep in mind that you don't want to create such incredibly high expectations of yourself and of the birth experience that you're bound to be let down. Try to build in room for flexibility in your conception of the ultimate birth. Your little one might not be following the same game plan as you, and last-minute strategy changes are often required. Fortunately, if you work on your birth plan now, you can build in allowances for complications and save yourself unnecessary angst later.

Childbirth Classes

Most childbirth seminars available through hospitals and birthing centers are called *prepared childbirth classes*. Taking place in a classroom setting and using lectures, audio-visuals, and floor exercises to get you ready for labor and delivery, prepared childbirth classes can focus on one, two, or more birth philosophies. They can vary in length from several months of

Saturdays to a 1-day seminar. While hospital policy will dictate a lot of what's covered, here's a general idea of what you will experience:

- **Commiseration.** You'll interact with other pregnant couples and demonstrate that misery (and joy) truly does love company.
- **Reality.** Through lecture and (in many cases) actual video footage, you'll get the full scoop on what really goes on in labor and delivery.
- **Guided tour.** If your class is at a birthing center or hospital, you will probably get a tour of the facilities and some basic instructions on when and where to show up when labor hits. The best part? The nursery window stop, of course.
- **Teamwork.** Your husband, partner, or labor coach will learn more about his role in this process, and you might even be given homework to try out techniques at home.
- **After-birth instruction.** Many classes offer valuable information on breastfeeding basics and baby care. Don't be surprised if the instructor brings in a bag full of baby dolls for practice.
- **Seasoned support.** Most prepared childbirth classes will be conducted by a trained childbirth educator.
- **Paperwork.** More literature, brochures, pamphlets, handouts, forms, photocopies, and leaflets will come your way. Bring a bag.

Perhaps the most important facet of childbirth class (and certainly the one that most first-time moms pay the closest attention to) is the information it provides on managing labor and delivery discomforts. In addition to an overview of anesthesia and pain medication options, childbirth educators draw on one or more childbirth philosophies to teach coping methods. Some of the most popular and widely taught techniques are outlined below.

Lamaze Method

Lamaze technique (psychoprophylaxis) is probably the most well-known childbirth method in use in the United States today. Named after Dr. Fernand Lamaze, classes are taught by certified Lamaze instructors and attended by more than two million parents-to-be annually.

Dr. Fernand Lamaze came up with the kernel of his theories on pain-less prepared childbirth after a trip to Russia in the early 1950s, a trip that familiarized him with the works of Ivan Pavlov. Pavlov was the Nobel-winning behavioral scientist behind the famed drooling dogs that were conditioned to equate the sound of a bell with their dinner.

If you've never been in a Lamaze class, you probably associate the name with heavy, hyperventilated breathing. True Lamaze classes, however, are much more than panting practice. Although rhythmic breathing exercises are stressed for each stage of labor in Lamaze, helpful laboring and birth positions, relaxation techniques, and pain management are also covered. In addition to massage, water therapy, and hot and cold compresses, you're taught how to focus on a picture or object to diminish your discomfort.

Lamaze is founded on the principal that instinct and what Lamaze International calls *inner wisdom* guide women through the birth process. Lamaze also stresses the empowerment of the mother-to-be and her right to the birth experience and environment she wants.

Bradley Method

Denver obstetrician Robert Bradley, author of *Husband-Coached Child-birth*, developed this popular approach to labor and delivery. As you may have guessed, he is a big advocate of fathers helping their partners through the birth process, and in fact many consider his work instrumental in open-ing up the labor room door to dads.

Bradley classes teach couples how to relax and breathe deeply, but the emphasis is on doing what comes naturally: father as coach, proper nutrition during pregnancy, and—most important—knowing all the options before-hand. They also emphasize the *natural* in natural childbirth, suggesting that pain medication be used as a last resort rather than as a frontline tool.

Hypnobirthing and Dr. Grantly Dick-Read

British doctor and natural childbirth pioneer Grantly Dick-Read, who authored the classic *Childbirth Without Fear*, is the inspiration behind hyp-nobirthing education. Dick-Read believes that a woman's labor pains are magnified by her fear and anxieties. Hypnobirthing, based on Dick-Read's teachings, emphasizes slow abdominal breathing and other relaxation techniques that teach you how to focus on the feelings and signals your body sends during labor.

Leboyer Method

Dr. Frederick Leboyer, author of *Birth Without Violence*, developed this method of childbirth that attempts to soften the trauma of the transition from the warm, dark womb to the big, bright world. It advocates dim lights in the delivery room, a warm bath for the new baby, calm voices, and soothing room temperatures.

The Right Teacher and the Right Class

Completely confused now? A good first step is to call your hospital or birthing center and ask for printed schedules and descriptions of upcoming classes; many of your questions will probably be answered right then. Once you get a basic feel for what is offered, you can call with follow-up questions about instructor credentials and training, methods taught, class sizes, curriculum, and costs. You might also ask if there are couples who have taken the course whom you can contact as references.

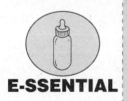

E-SSENTIAL

If you've had a previous cesarean section, ask about a VBAC class, which provides couples with information on the benefits, risks, and statistics surrounding vaginal births following a cesarean section. It is usually recommended as a supplement to, rather than a replacement for, a prepared childbirth class.

If you find that the classes or curriculum offered at your local hospital just aren't what you're looking for, you can opt for private instruction. The International Childbirth Education Association (ICEA) will provide you with names of certified instructors in your area. You can contact ICEA at 800-624-4934 or online at *www.icea.org*.

Touring the Hospital/Birthing Center

Even if you don't choose a childbirth class sponsored by the facility at which you'll be giving birth, you should try to arrange a tour. Getting your bearings ahead of time will save you valuable time and frustration when the big day arrives. When you're in the middle of the mother-of-all contractions, the last thing you want to do is try to figure out where validated parking is. You'll also have less anxiety and disappointment if you know what to expect of the labor and birthing rooms. What you imagine (a flower-filled, sunny room filled with soft music and framed watercolors) may be a far cry from reality.

Classes for Siblings

New-sibling classes can be a huge boon for parents who are on their second pregnancy. Typically divided by age group so that information can be communicated at an appropriate level, these classes put an emphasis on the emotional side of having a new family member—how things at home are changing, how the family will adjust after baby is born, and what the children are feeling about these developments.

E-QUESTION

The childbirth educator asked if we had a pediatrician. Isn't it too early?
Your pediatrician will care for your newborn in the hospital, so getting one lined up now is important. Some things to inquire about: Are lactation consultants available? How are phone calls triaged and returned? Do ill children have a separate waiting room?

There's also plenty of practical information provided, including a preview tour of mom's accommodations and some basic big-sibling guidelines for baby handling. Even the youngest kids are usually given the opportunity to practice baby care with a doll.

If your child is having difficulty adjusting to the idea of a new baby in the house, a sibling class can make him feel more involved in, and consequently more accepting of, your family's growth. As you might imagine, the ability of the instructor to relate to your child can make or break this type of class, so getting a few referrals is time well spent. If you have the opportunity, you might inquire about the possibility of spending 15 minutes in the back of an upcoming class to test the waters before sending your child to participate.

Just for Dads

Depending on today's viewpoint, the light or the fire at the end of the tunnel is becoming brighter. In 3 months you will be witnessing your child's first breath in this world. Although your partner will be doing the grunt work, you'll need to start studying your role in this final drama as (1) a shoulder to lean on; (2) a forgiving target to vent at; and (3) head cheerleader.

About Childbirth Classes

If you are the type who thrives on clear instructions and routine, you might find the idea of childbirth class a port in the pregnancy storm. "Woo hoo!" you think. "At last someone is going to tell me what to do." Well, not quite. Yes, you will be taught techniques you can use to help your partner through labor and delivery, and you'll learn in graphic detail just how that baby is going to get from point A to point B. But you aren't receiving any step-by-step instructions or checklists that are money-back guaranteed to get you from the first contraction to "It's a boy/girl!" Labor and delivery are not a math problem or a computer program. Your best preparation is to be ready for the unexpected.

Don't think of class as . . . well, class, either. It is an educational experience, although you aren't being graded on your perfor-mance. In other words, if academics are not your strong suit, you don't need to be in a panic. The only background you need to succeed in childbirth class is a willing-ness to learn and listen—and a preg-nant partner. There will be no pop quizzes there.

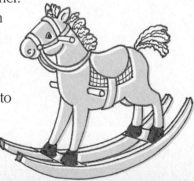

E-FACT

Second, third, or fourth time around? There are benefits to taking a childbirth class for even the most experienced parents. If there's something new under the sun in labor and delivery, class is the place to learn about it. Many facilities also offer special brush-up courses for veterans of the pregnancy wars.

Coaching lesson number one: think little league, not major league baseball. Coaching means being supportive, helping your "rookie" learn the game of birth as she progresses through labor, giving her the tools she needs to get through the rough spots, and—above all—providing positive reinforcement and encouragement.

Blueprint for Birth: Writing Your Birth Plan

A birth plan is a road map for your entire childbirth experience, beginning to end. It's your chance to let everyone involved (doctors, nurses, partners) know what you want the experience to be. Anything you have definitive expectations about should be outlined in your birth plan, from your wishes regarding pain relief to specifications for how your newborn is fed and cared for in the hospital. Use it to chart the course of labor and delivery, but remember that you might have to take alternate routes occasionally depending on conditions.

Why Have a Birth Plan?

The process of talking through and creating a birth plan helps you and your partner establish what you want out of childbirth (aside from the child, of course). Having it down as written word can ease your anxieties about labor and delivery. And when things get crazy as the big day arrives, a birth plan can be your calm in the storm, something solid to grasp when you suddenly seem to have forgotten just about everything you've learned.

A birth plan also serves the very important purpose of letting your provider know just what kind of experience and what level of interventions you're looking for. Because the plan can tread on some sensitive and controversial medical territory, it's important that you include your doctor or midwife in the process.

Preparing Your Provider

Once you and your partner have your birth plan together, you should present it to your provider for his comments and questions. Communicating your wishes and being receptive to feedback can make the difference between a birth plan that works and one that doesn't.

Many physicians and midwives will set up a separate office visit dedicated to discussing the birth plan you've come up with. Consider the plan you initially take to her to be a first draft. You can then incorporate your provider's input into your final plan.

Unfortunately, not all practitioners are thrilled about the prospect of a birth plan. This can be a hot-button issue for physicians who either feel as if their patients don't trust them or don't want to have a disappointed patient if the actual birth strays from the plan. For these reasons, birth plans have the potential to set up an adversarial situation in some doctor-patient relationships.

How can you prevent your birth plan from becoming a bone of contention? First, be willing to really listen to any suggestions or issues your provider has and make an effort to work toward a resolution together. Also, try to keep your expectations grounded in reality and not overly restrictive. Wanting your three-year-old to be nearby so that she can meet her sibling shortly after birth is great, but insisting she be front and center the moment baby's head emerges is unrealistic.

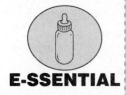

Once you have reviewed your birth plan with your practitioner and made your final changes, ask him to place a copy in your chart and hospital record. Make sure your labor coach and other support people who will be present at the birth have one as well, so everyone is playing by the same game plan.

Make It User Friendly

If you hand your doctor a birth plan the size of *War and Peace*, she might start to wonder what she's gotten herself into. While covering all your bases is important, you simply can't control every possible aspect of what does or doesn't occur during labor and delivery. Medical emergencies do happen, which is why you have signed on a practitioner to begin with. You need to trust your provider to follow the spirit of your birth plan while making adjustments for your health and that of your baby. Establishing a good communicative relationship is the best way to ensure this.

Conciseness is better from a logistical viewpoint, too. The medical staff attending your birth and aftercare should be able to easily access and reference the information. Think brevity and bullet points—the CliffsNotes of your thoughts on how you'd like birth to proceed. Keep the plan under five pages, if possible; fewer than that is even better.

Try to use language that is cooperative and communicative. Your birth plan should not read like a ransom note. Filling it with demands and absolutes leaves your provider very little room to make appropriate medical suggestions should birth go off course.

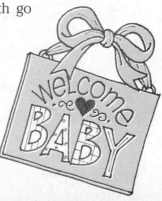

The bottom line is that labor is very unpredictable and rarely do birth plans get followed to the letter. Outlining your wishes in terms of preferences and giving your provider alternatives in case complications arise will make your birth plan more useful to everyone involved, especially to you and baby.

Atmosphere

Comfortable surroundings will help both your mind and body relax during labor. Whether you're giving birth in a hospital, at home, or somewhere in between, outlining your preference for what you'll be seeing and hearing around you is an important component of the birth plan.

The Perfect Place

First, know what you have to work with. Hospital birthing facilities are starting to recognize the value of a homey, warm atmosphere. You may find that yours is already set up to suit your needs well.

However, if the setting looks a little sterile and Spartan, there are ways to make it more welcoming. Easy and acceptable additions include a cozy blanket and pillow from home, a picture or two (which can serve double duty as focal points during contractions), and fresh flowers. You might also be able to adjust the lights and sounds to make the environment more relaxing.

Home birth is an option if you feel strongly about giving birth in familiar surroundings and among family. However, home birth doesn't mean you should opt out of a health care professional's help; in fact, this is even more important since you won't have access to the medical monitoring and diagnostic equipment that a hospital offers. In many uncomplicated pregnancies, a home birth can be a completely safe and emotionally rewarding choice. However, women who might experience high-risk deliveries for any reason need to seriously contemplate the benefits and safety of a hospital birth.

E-ALERT!

Be aware that professional and insurance restrictions may prohibit your doctor from attending a home birth. If your provider can't be there and your mind is set on a home birth, find out if he can refer you to a midwife or doctor who can attend.

An in-between alternative for some women is a birthing center, which is equipped to handle some medical problems that may occur yet can offer some less conventional laboring and delivery methods, such as a water birth.

Music and Lighting

Music is one of the easiest ways to change the mood. Just bring a portable stereo and a few diverse musical selections, in case you need a change of pace, and you're all set. Classical music can help to soothe and center you, while something fast and furious can get the adrenaline going for the hard work. Just be conscious of the fact that other moms will likely be laboring nearby and that your baby is not wearing earplugs. Keep the volume down, or use headphones if you don't mind yet another line hooking you up.

As far as lighting goes, you might not have a lot of choices beyond off/on if you're giving birth in a hospital setting. Even if you can dim the lights, you want your provider to be able to see what she's doing. But requesting that the drapes be drawn and the lights be turned down during early and active labor is not unreasonable.

Photo Finish

Chances are you will want pictures, and lots of them. Your birth plan can outline your audiovisual expectations (for example, video of the delivery, pictures of a C-section in the operating room, live webcast of baby's first breath). The plan also serves as a good checklist for you and your partner when packing for the hospital.

If you want to capture your little star's debut on video, it's best to check with your provider to make sure there's no policy against an amateur videographer being underfoot. Even if there is, in some cases you might be able to work out a compromise, such as setting up the camera in advance on a stationary tripod.

Family, Friends, and Support

So, who will be at the big event? This is perhaps one of the most crucial parts of a birth plan: to prepare for adequate support during this very difficult job that lies ahead. Is this a personal experience for just your partner and you, or do you want additional family, friends, or doula support there? The decision is even tougher for first-time moms, who may have some misconceptions about exactly what will happen and who will be there when they hit the maternity ward.

Many women think that their provider or, at the least, a dedicated staff nurse will be available to assist them with the entire labor and birth. In most places that simply isn't true, for a variety of reasons. Shift changes, the number of patients in labor, and other factors may have you and your partner spending a lot of the time alone. Having a doula on your labor team is a great way to ensure continuity of care.

Why enlist a doula's assistance if a dad or coach is present? Many doulas will provide early labor support at home, a benefit that most practitioners can't match. It's also reassuring to many dads to know that they have a backup and aren't forced to remember everything they learned in their 6-week childbirth class during this emotionally charged time.

If you will have people waiting at the hospital who won't be participating in your birth but whom you would like to introduce to the baby as soon after delivery as possible, indicate your wishes in the birth plan. And don't forget about a caregiver for any younger children present, who will need supervision and support.

Getting Ready

You have the people and the place set. Now for some decisions that will affect your comfort and mobility during labor.

Labor Prep Preferences

Shaving, enemas, and intravenous lines are just a few of the ways the nursing staff may get you ready for the rest of your labor and for delivery. You have the option of doing some of these steps yourself and foregoing others completely. Whatever you decide, make it a part of your birth plan.

Food and Drink

Some hospitals and providers put a strict ban on lunching during labor, for several reasons. First, if events don't go as planned and you end up having to have a general anesthetic for a C-section, having food in your stomach puts you at risk for aspiration (inhaling vomit). Second, your stomach and gastrointestinal tract will have to digest that food when clearly there is more important action happening right next door.

E-ALERT!

That said, labor is a marathon that lasts exceedingly long for many women, who may need some sustenance to make it through. Simple, liquid-based carbohydrates such as a glass of juice, a Popsicle or juice bar, broth, or tea or lemonade with honey are easily digested and can give you the boost you need. Outline what you'd like to have access to so that you can discuss it with your doctor. If your provider or hospital believes a light snack of food and drink is an absolute no-no in labor, intravenous lines will probably be used to take care of any risk of dehydration. However, a dry mouth is annoying and uncomfortable, so see if you can at least get ice chips to suck on, and bring your lip balm.

Monitors and Mobility

Being tethered to a bed can make handling contractions and labor difficult. Yet checking the fetal heart rate and your contractions is important to ensure that baby isn't encountering any stress. To give yourself room to move through the contractions while ensuring your little one's safety, ask for intermittent monitoring. Unless you require internal monitoring, which is sometimes the case in higher-risk pregnancies, having the freedom to move at least part of the time shouldn't be an issue. Wireless fetal monitors can let you cut the cord altogether; ask your hospital or birthing center if they use them.

Pain Relief

One of the biggest decisions of childbirth is whether you will want or need pharmaceutical pain relief. Your provider and anesthesiologist can also shed more light on the use of painkillers if you have additional questions.

Going Natural

If you intend to go completely drug free, this section of your birth plan will be a bit more detailed than others. You'll want to outline the access you'd like to drug-free pain relief strategies. Practices like hydrotherapy (shower or whirlpool), massage, and birth balls might be on your list. Requesting to go natural doesn't close the door on changing your mind. If you're a first-time mom, you can't predict whether or not pain medication will be necessary.

Timing of Pain Relief

Some practitioners have policies about how late (or how early) in labor they will permit an epidural (an injection of drugs into the spinal column that decreases pain in the lower half of the body). Whether her policy is grounded in research, experience, or preference will probably make the difference in whether your provider is willing to be flexible on this point. If you have strong feelings about when you want access to an epidural or other pain relief option, outline your wishes in your birth plan.

E-FACT

A birth ball is a large, inflatable rubber ball that you can sit on, drape yourself over, or do just about anything else that feels comfortable during a contraction. It is available in different sizes and in oblong or ridged versions for more stability. When used in the sitting position, the natural give of the ball encourages perineal relaxation.

When to Change Course: Interventions

Your doctor will warn you up front that unforeseen circumstances will mean a deviation from your birth plan. Sometimes women feel as if they have failed if matters do not go precisely according to their concept of the ideal birth—which is certainly not realistic. The best way to avoid disappointment is to build alternative scenarios into your birth plan regarding interventions that might be required. For example, if you really don't want an episiotomy (an incision between the vagina and the anus performed to widen the birth canal), you should indicate that in your birth plan and suggest perineal massage with vitamin E oil or another lubricant, warm compresses, or another acceptable alternative. But be prepared to work with your doctor during labor if your alternative plan just doesn't do the trick. And don't be too prescriptive—when you start instructing your physician in the type of sutures to use, you're forgetting that you've hired her because of her medical expertise, not in spite of it.

Some possible interventions that come up in labor and delivery include:

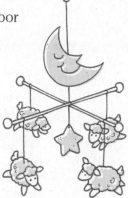

- Induction
- Forceps use
- Vacuum extraction
- Episiotomy
- Artificial membrane rupture

Other Considerations

The choices continue after labor and delivery and include decisions not just about your own care, but also about the care of your new son or daughter.

Cutting the Cord

You or your partner will probably be given the option to cut the baby's umbilical cord if you want to. Keep in mind that if your baby needs immediate medical attention at birth, it's possible the cord will be cut swiftly by the attending doctor or midwife instead.

The issue of when exactly to cut the cord could require some negotiations if you have strong feelings about delaying it. If your provider disagrees and believes a swift snip is in order, find out the reasons and research behind his opinion so that you can explore the issue further and come to a meeting of the minds, if possible.

First Contact

Every woman wants her first encounter with her baby to be just perfect. After all, you've had a 9-month buildup to this moment, so wanting to stage and execute it seamlessly is natural.

I'm having a C-section. Why bother with a birth plan?
Even with a cesarean birth, there are many choices along the way. Will dad cut the cord? Can video be taken? Will you get to hold your baby right after the procedure? A birth plan will help you clarify these issues with your doctor ahead of time.

If you're giving birth in a hospital, find out whether there are strict procedures that must be followed with the baby's care immediately following the birth. Will you be able to nuzzle with her for as long as you'd like, or will she be whisked away for cleaning, fingerprinting, and the rest after a quick hello? Will your other children be able to meet her immediately, or will they have to wait until visiting hours? Contact your birth facility before you create this part of your plan so that you aren't in for an immediate letdown if your wishes for the first encounter are against hospital policy. If you find the policies are just too restrictive, you still have time to explore other options for where you deliver.

Creative thinking may be required to make some rules and regulations acceptable to you. If you can only hold your baby for a few minutes before she goes for her after-birth tune-up, perhaps your partner can assist with those duties and use this special time to bond with baby himself.

Rooming In or Out

Do you want baby to spend just about every waking moment within arm's reach, or will you need some time to catch up on your vast sleep deficit? If you prefer the former, having baby spend days and particularly nights in your room with you, a setup called *rooming in*, should be included in your birth plan.

I don't want my baby getting a bottle in the hospital. Should I put this in the birth plan?
Definitely. Even though the nursing staff usually asks about feeding preferences, if you're planning on breastfeeding and want to ensure that your baby establishes a good technique in those early days, it's wise to note your preferences in your birth plan.

Again, how much time baby sleeps with you or in the nursery may be a matter of hospital policy. However, given what research has uncovered about the importance of early bonding and nurturing and the emphasis on establishing milk supply for breastfeeding moms, it's fairly uncommon to find a facility that won't give you the choice of having your baby in the room with you. In general, you should be able to have your little one with you as much as you'd like. And if you need a short nap and the baby is not tired, the nursing staff is always there as backup.

Postpartum Planning

Adding a postpartum section to your birth plan can be a tremendous help in getting organized after you and your baby are back at home. Will you have live-in help for a few days or weeks? Are you and your partner both taking time off? Will baby have a whirlwind schedule of introductions to friends and family or just a few exclusive engagements?

Outline your maternity leave timetable, if you know what it is, and tentative plans after it's over. Include baby's 2-week doctor visit so that you won't forget to schedule it when she arrives.

Even though your health care provider won't need to put his stamp of approval on this portion of your plan, it's a good idea to run this by him. He can give you feedback on whether you'll be physically capable of doing what you've set out to do in order to ensure that you have a sufficient recovery period.

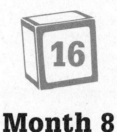

Month 8

You are a pregnancy pro now, deftly handling all the aches and pains that come with the territory. Even if you're one of the lucky ones who sail through pregnancy feeling just fine, you've still faced down plenty of lifestyle challenges by now. You have learned to adjust to the fashion hardships, the changes in your home and routine, and the logistical struggles that your baby and belly have brought to the forefront. It's not much longer now.

Baby This Month

Gradually shifting to the position in which approximately 95 percent of all babies are born, your fetus starts to move into a head-down pose, known as the *vertex position*. The small but stubborn percentage that don't assume the vertex position are considered breech. Feel a lot of kicking on your pelvic floor? It could be a clue that baby is still standing or sitting tall. She might also be lounging in the transverse (sideways) position in the womb.

Your little one is now up to 18 inches long and as heavy as a 5-pound sack of flour. The rest of her body is finally catching up to the size of her head. Although it may feel like she's constantly up and about, she's actually sleeping 90 to 95 percent of the day, a figure that will drop only slightly when she is born.

If your child were born today, she'd have an excellent chance of surviving and eventually thriving outside the womb. However, she'd still be considered preterm or premature, as is any birth before week 37 of gestation.

Your Body This Month

Can you still remember your prepregnancy body? The little things—like being able to zip up your coat, wear your rings, and sit on the floor without requiring adult assistance to stand again—may be a distant memory. You will not be pregnant forever, of course, although it might sometimes feel that way.

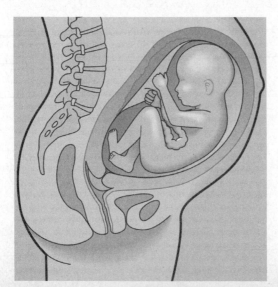

You and your baby in the 8th month of gestation

208

Your Body Changes

Weight gain should start to slow down this month. If it doesn't, however, don't cut your calorie intake below 2,600 to try to stop it. You need the extra energy for both of you.

As baby settles firmly on your bladder, bathroom stops step up once again. You may even experience some stress incontinence: minor dribbling or leakage of urine when you sneeze, cough, laugh, or make other sudden movements. This will clear up postpartum. In the meantime, keep doing your Kegels, don't hold it in, and wear a panty liner.

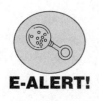

E-ALERT!

Amniotic fluid is clear to straw-colored and has a faintly sweet smell. Less commonly, it may be tinged green or brown. If you think you're leaking amniotic fluid, no matter how small the amount, contact your care provider. If your membranes have ruptured, you risk infection if you don't deliver soon.

What You Feel Like

Your Weeble-like physique has you off balance and generally klutzy. Be careful: You wobble, and you can fall down. And, of course, those (say it together, everyone) pregnancy hormones have loosened up your joints and relaxed your muscles to make you a bit of a butterfingers.

Now is not the ideal time to be fitted for new contacts or glasses. Pregnancy-related fluid retention can actually change the shape of your eyes and trigger minor vision changes. Also at work is estrogen, which causes your eyes to be drier than normal and can make contact lenses uncomfortable right now. Unless you want to invest in new eyewear again postpartum, you should hold off on any such purchase for now.

Although you may not relish the thought of air travel in your current wide-body state, for most women in low-risk pregnancies, flying is safe through week 36. Obviously, if something happens while you are in the air or away from home, you would need to get care from providers you don't know, and that can be very stressful. If you do need to fly late in your pregnancy, consider taking a copy of your prenatal chart in case any problems do arise.

Some airlines restrict air travel after a certain point in pregnancy because they don't want to deal with any complications, while others require a doctor's note for travel. Check with individual airlines regarding their policies when booking your flight.

Dehydration due to the low humidity in airplane cabins can be avoided by drinking fluids during the flight. Skip the soda and stick with water or juice; the low air pressure in the cabin also makes gas expand and can make carbonated beverages and other gas-producing foods an uncomfortable choice.

There is a theoretical concern about developing blood clots while immobilized on a flight, but this has not been well documented; moving around in your seat and walking to the bathroom will probably be enough to prevent their occurrence.

It's increasingly easy to get winded as your little one pushes up into your diaphragm. Take it slow, breathe deeply, and practice good posture. To ease breathing while you sleep, pile on a few extra pillows or use a foam bed wedge to elevate your head.

Other symptoms that may continue this month include:

✓ Fatigue
✓ Frequent urination
✓ Tender and/or swollen breasts
✓ Colostrum discharge from nipples
✓ Bleeding gums
✓ Excess mucus and saliva
✓ Increase in normal vaginal discharge
✓ Mild shortness of breath
✓ Lightheadedness or dizziness
✓ Headaches
✓ Forgetfulness
✓ Gas, heartburn, and/or constipation
✓ Skin and hair changes
✓ Round ligament pain or soreness
✓ Lower-back aches
✓ Mild swelling of legs, feet, and hands
✓ Leg cramps
✓ Painless, irregular contractions (Braxton-Hicks)

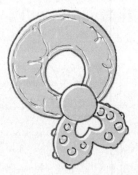

If you experience blurry vision or visual disturbances (for example, spots), let your provider know immediately. Either one could be a sign of high blood pressure, which is dangerous to both you and your child. These are also symptoms of preeclampsia, which can be dangerous for both you and your baby.

At Your Doctor Visit

You'll see your provider twice or more this month as you continue your every-other-week routine. She will check the position of your baby to determine whether he has turned head down in preparation for birth.

If your practitioner brings up the possibility of a breech birth (bottom- or foot-first), it's because she has felt the head of your unborn baby up near your ribs, or an ultrasound has confirmed that your child is in the breech position. Don't panic. Your fickle fetus is likely to change position again in the next few weeks. If she doesn't, your practitioner may try to turn the baby once you're closer to term, using a technique known as *external cephalic version*: manually attempting to turn the fetus in the uterus. ACOG recommends that an external cephalic version be attempted in most breech cases, typically between weeks 36 and 42.

E-FACT

External cephalic version (or simply *version*) is successful in turning a breech baby in about half of all instances where it is attempted. However, if it is done too far in advance of the estimated delivery date, there is a possibility that the fetus may flip back to the breech position.

Babies can be delivered vaginally in breech position in some instances, but the procedure is more difficult and carries a higher risk for the infant. If your provider has not been adequately trained to perform vaginal breech delivery (and many are no longer so trained), you could be offered a C-section. Currently, C-section is the method of choice for a safe breech delivery. If you really want a vaginal birth and a cephalic version is unsuccessful in turning your breech, some practitioners may agree to a trial of labor to see if your contracting uterus helps to turn the child.

There are three classifications of breech: frank, complete, and incomplete. In frank breech, your baby uses your pelvic bone as a seat and stretches his legs up close to his chest. In a complete breech, your baby has his bottom on your pelvis again, but legs and arms are crossed in front of his little body. A footling breech is not a good candidate for vaginal delivery because the diameter of the legs will be smaller than the head, resulting in an increased risk of entrapment (the head being too large to move through the cervix). With incomplete breech, one or both legs will drop down during delivery and will arrive before the rest of the body. This is also called a *single- or double-footling breech birth.*

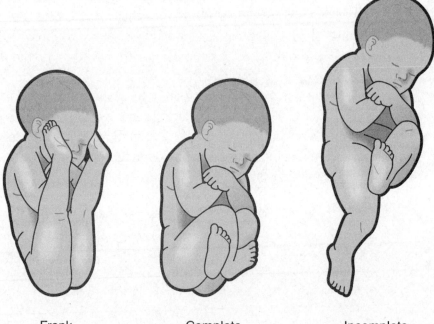

Frank   Complete   Incomplete

There are three classifications of breech: frank, complete, and incomplete.

On Your Mind

As labor looms closer, your thoughts turn to the task at hand. Going into labor and delivery with as much knowledge of the process as possible can make the difference between a positive childbirth experience and a long and arduous one.

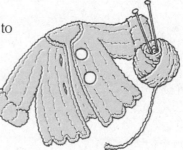

"Am I Up To the Task of Labor?"

Women have been doing this since the beginning of time and under much more difficult circumstances. Yes, in most cases labor will be hard work, but if you prepare yourself by learning what to expect, you will be ready to face whatever comes your way. You'll also find that your spouse or labor partner and coach will be a huge asset in helping you through childbirth.

"Am I Up To the Task of Motherhood?"

Great mommies are made, not born. Although some aspects of mothering will seem to come to you instinctively, practice and trial and error will make up the better part of your parenting education. Use the tools around you—your pediatrician, other mothers, and research and reading—to build and sharpen your skills. In the final analysis, listen to your inner voice in the application of what you learn.

Things That Make You Go Grrrrr

As pregnancy winds down, your patience goes with it. The belly rubbers, advice givers, urban-legend spreaders, and comedians seem to be everywhere and completely unaware of the dangerously thin ice they are treading on. Rather than biting heads off, take a deep, deep breath and remind yourself that though insensitive, most are well meaning. In the meantime, photocopy the following list of no-nos for your coworkers and hang it in the break room; maybe it will sink in.

E-QUESTION

What if I don't get to the hospital in time?
The average labor lasts 12 to 14 hours, plenty of time to get to the hospital. To avoid any unforeseen delays, work out a route in advance, keep your gas tank full, and have cash on hand for a cab in case your car conks out with the first contraction.

Top ten things not to say to a pregnant woman:

1. Haven't you had that baby yet?
2. Are you still here?
3. Wow, you're HUGE!
4. You really should avoid pain medication when you go into labor; it will hurt the baby.
5. Labor is hell! Take all the drugs you can get!
6. So, how much weight have you gained?
7. You don't mind if we call you at home while you're on maternity leave, do you?
8. Are you having twins?
9. You look terrible; why don't you take a nap?
10. Sorry—our restrooms are for employees only.

Bed Rest

If you're experiencing a medical condition that puts you at risk for preterm labor, your provider may send you to your room—for strict bed rest. Bed rest takes the forces of gravity off your cervix, gives your circulatory system and blood pressure a break, and has the added benefit of promoting rest and stress reduction.

Staying Sane

At first that bed may seem like a welcome oasis, particularly if you've been getting little sleep as of late. A prescription to snooze! What more could you ask for?

That feeling will likely be short-lived, however. There's only so much you can do horizontally (or even slightly tilted). Yet there are ways to make the time pass a little faster. Some ideas to keep busy beyond the usual TV and movie fare:

- **Baby shopping by mail or web.** Get on your laptop or leaf through some of those catalogs your mailbox has been inundated with. Shopping has never been so easy on your feet.
- **Get crafty.** Creating something special for baby—embroidered, crocheted, or knitted—is a good way to pass the hours. Even if you are a rookie, a beginner's kit can get you started. You may not have the time again for years, so go for it.
- **Feed your mind.** Read, read, read. Not just baby books (although feel free to keep this one handy), but classics, new fiction, and anything else you can get your hands on.
- **Catch up.** All those pictures you've been meaning to put into photo albums, the scrapbooks that are half finished, letters on your list to write, and other assorted undertakings are perfect bed rest projects that have the added bonus of imparting a sense of achievement.
- **Be game.** Dust off some of those old board and strategy games you haven't played in years, and recruit your partner or kids to play, too. A rousing game of Risk can be a lot more entertaining than another evening spent channel surfing.

Nesting

Ah, nesting—that overwhelming urge to turn everything in your house upside down and rearrange it just so. Your mad dash to finish the nursery and squirrel away a year's supply of diaper wipes is an instinctive reaction to baby's upcoming arrival. You're preparing a safe haven for your little one and assuring yourself that all his needs and wants will be adequately met.

A Space for Baby the First Few Weeks

Keeping baby within arm's length during her first few weeks home will improve your rest and peace of mind. A bassinet, about the size and depth of a baby carriage or pram, can make her feel safer and more secure than in the open space of a crib, after spending 9 months in close quarters. And you can roll a bassinet right next to your bed to give those 4 A.M. feedings with ease. It's also an inexpensive way to bunk her down if you're still saving your pennies for the perfect crib.

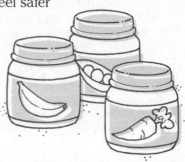

Stocking Up on Essentials

Don't go crazy buying supersized cases of baby supplies. You may not like the brand or configuration you purchase, which leaves you with a lot of unwanted merchandise on your hands. Instead, buy small so that you can sample. Once you've decided what works best for you and baby, you can stock up at the warehouse store.

And now is the time to start thinking about whether you want to go cloth or disposable with diapers. If you're thinking green, cloth diapers have the advantage of not ending up in a landfill, although they do require additional fossil fuels and water resources to wash and transport (if you use a service). Cost can be an advantage, but it's probably a slight one if you use a service. Call local diaper services to get estimates and a rundown of what's included. You can wash them at home, of course, but be sure you have the time and the strength to be doing laundry daily. If your baby has sensitive skin, you might find cloth less irritating. Like most things in parenting, it's trial and error; have a supply of both and see how each works for you.

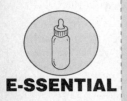

E-SSENTIAL

Some baby essentials you should have on hand prior to her arrival: diapers (of course), wipes, alcohol swabs (for her umbilical cord), baby shampoo and soap, diaper-rash ointment, waterproof pads (a huge plus for cutting down on laundry), bottles (even if you're breastfeeding you might pump milk), a thermometer, and a fever-reducing product (for example, Tylenol) recommended by your pediatrician.

Just for Dads

Indecision and insecurities may plague you this month as the birth draws nearer, made all the more disturbing by any unfamiliarity with these feelings. Try to conquer any anxieties you may have by accepting your weaknesses and valuing your strengths. And recognize the fact that learning is all part of the experience.

Measuring Up

Whether you aspire to be just like your father or have sworn to be nothing like him at all, you've got some preconceived notion of just what makes the world's best dad. Beyond your own childhood, your idea of fatherhood has been shaped by many different influences, not the least of which are the impossibly patient patriarchs dramatized on the small screen. But though they're nice to watch, you wouldn't want to live with them. Don't try to measure up to a fantasy figure.

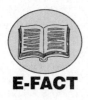

E-FACT

Trying to break the baby-name stalemate? If you are set on one name and your partner on another, consider combinations of the two or variations with first and middle names. Still not agreeing? Start from scratch and find something that you both like. Be sure to consider all possible nicknames, initials, and obvious rhyming combinations to spare your child later grief.

Start with the basics. Promise yourself you'll listen to your child, be there for him, and instill a sense of values and moral compass through your actions and your words. Love him. That's what a father does best.

Diaper Duty and Other Special Skills

If you're a complete novice at infant care, the best way to pick up pointers is to take a baby care class at your local hospital. You may feel silly playing with dolls at first, but when you do it in a room full of other grown men following suit, it's easier to take. However, if a class isn't an option for you, and you don't have any babies of family or friends that you can take for a test drive, it won't take you long to learn once your baby arrives.

You'll have the opportunity to diaper your newborn during her stay in the hospital, under the watchful eye of a nurse if you so desire. This is a safe environment in which to learn if you're a little wary of your abilities. Take advantage of it.

The first bath is always cause for some jitters, but your newborn won't be having anything beyond a sponging off until she's back at home and her cord has fallen off (yes, it's supposed to do that). Tag teaming with your partner on the baby bathing is a great approach to take until you've built up your confidence level.

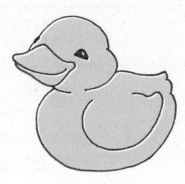

Month 9

You've finally reached the final weeks of pregnancy, and the grand finale is approaching. You probably feel like you've been waiting forever. But even if you're sure you have the time of conception pinpointed, your baby may decide he needs a little more time preparing (or a little less). This is your first lesson in parental patience. Try not to hold him too closely to your schedule; he will arrive, sooner or later.

Baby This Month

Your child is packing on about a half-pound per week as he prepares to make his big exit. He's fully formed and just waiting for the right time now. If you're having a boy, his testicles have descended and may be visible in any 9-month ultrasound images. His lungs, the last organ system to fully mature, now have an adequate level of surfactant in them to allow breathing outside the womb.

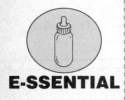

E-SSENTIAL

A pregnancy is considered full-term from weeks 37 to 42. Only 5 percent of expectant women actually give birth on their estimated date of delivery, and first-time moms are more likely to go past their due date. If you've delivered a baby before, however, statistically you are more likely to give birth within 4 days of your EDD.

A dark, tarry amalgam of amniotic fluid, skin cells, and other fetal waste is gathering in your baby's intestines. This substance (called *meconium*) will become the contents of his bowel movements during the first few days of life.

Fetal movement will naturally slow down as you get closer to your due date and the baby is pressed for space, but a healthy baby should still be making his presence known. Your provider may ask you to count fetal kicks. Pick a typically active time of day for your little one, and start counting his moves. Your provider will let you know how many movements you should feel in what period of time (usually around eight to ten in a space of 2 hours).

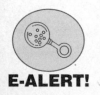

E-ALERT!

If your baby's movements aren't as frequent as your provider has told you they should be, it's possible she is sleeping. Try drinking a glass of juice to get her going. Be sure to call your provider immediately if fetal movements are notably decreased or absent.

Your Body This Month

While baby is still growing, your weight gain tapers off this month. Groin soreness and backaches are more persistent as the musculoskeletal system strains to support your abdomen. The good news: you can't get any bigger.

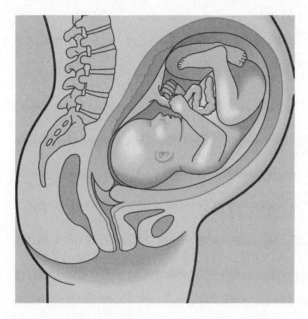

A final look at you and your fetus before the big day

Your Body Changes

Engagement (lightening), the process of the baby dropping down into the pelvic cavity in preparation for delivery, can occur any time now. In some women (particularly those who have given birth before), it may not happen until labor starts.

Your cervix is ripening (softening) in preparation for baby's passage. As it effaces (thins) and dilates (opens), the soft plug of mucus keeping it sealed tight may be dislodged. This mass, with the appealing name of *mucous plug*, may be tinged red or pink; it is also referred to by the equally explicit *bloody show*.

What You Feel Like

If the baby has dropped, you could be running to the bathroom more than ever. He also may be sending shockwaves through your pelvis as he settles further down onto the pelvic floor. On the up side, you can finally breathe as he pulls away from your lungs and diaphragm. Braxton-Hicks contractions can be more frequent this month as you draw nearer to delivery. You're close enough to be on the lookout for the real things, however. How will you recognize them?

Real contractions will:

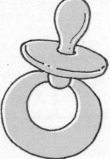

- ✓ Be felt in the back and possibly radiate around to the abdomen.
- ✓ Not subside when you move around or change positions.
- ✓ Increase in intensity as time passes.
- ✓ Come at roughly regular intervals (early on, this can be from 20 to 45 minutes apart).
- ✓ Increase in intensity with activities like walking.

Other signs that labor is on its way include amniotic fluid that leaks in either a gush or a trickle (your "water breaking"), sudden diarrhea, and the appearance of the mucous plug. Keep in mind, however, that for many women, the bag of waters does not break until active labor sets in.

At Your Doctor Visit

You'll see your doctor on a weekly basis from now until you deliver. Unless you are scheduled for a planned cesarean, your provider will probably perform an internal exam with each visit to check your cervix for changes that indicate approaching labor.

Tests This Month

The CDC recommends that your provider administer a group B strep (GBS) test in weeks 35 to 37. This culture is performed by swabbing a sample from both your vagina and your rectum. If the cultured sample comes back positive for GBS, you may have intravenous antibiotics administered during delivery to prevent group B strep bacteria transmission to the baby.

Checking Your Cervix

Your provider will be checking your cervix for signs that it is preparing for your baby's passage. She'll also be taking note of any descent or dropping of the baby toward the pelvis, called the *station*. Take the numbers you hear with a grain of salt, however. Although you may start effacing and dilating now, it's still anyone's guess as to when labor will begin, and it could be a few more weeks yet.

On Your Mind

You're likely tired but happy as you pack and prepare for the big day. Just remember the "estimated" in "estimated delivery date" to avoid a big letdown if baby is tardy.

Tired of Being Pregnant

You are so ready to have this baby. Nothing fits, not even your shoes. You can't sleep for more than a few hours at a time. Your belly itches and your breasts ache. You look toward your due date like a long distance runner approaching the end of a marathon. As you waddle toward the finish line, enjoy these final sensations of your child moving inside of you—the funny little hiccups, the elbow and knee bumps parading across your belly, and the subtle nudges that remind you you're not alone even if no one else is around.

When your cervix hasn't budged and your due date has come and gone, you may be tempted to try one of those sure-fire homemade labor inducers that every pregnant woman hears about. Castor oil, herbal concoctions, spicy food, breast massage, and sex are just a few methods bandied about in pregnancy chatrooms everywhere.

Unfortunately, some "natural methods" might only succeed in making you nauseated, while others can pose a real danger. Even if you're embarrassed, you need to run these by your doctor or midwife before taking matters into your own hands. A good provider will listen and won't laugh, letting you know what's safe and what isn't.

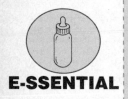

Massaging the areola and gently rolling the nipple mimics the action of a nursing baby and stimulates the natural release of oxytocin, which triggers uterine contractions. Several clinical studies have shown that this method can be useful in labor induction and also helpful in reducing postpartum hemorrhage.

Irritable and Anxious

As sleep gets more and more elusive and your discomfort ratchets up, you may find yourself easily provoked. The best short-term solution to keeping your cool? Stay clear of encounters with people you just know will irritate you (whether they mean to or not), and ask your significant other to be the point person on all those "Anything yet?" questions.

First-time moms may find themselves overwhelmed with anxiety now that birth is so near. Take a deep breath, go over what you learned in childbirth class (repeatedly, if it helps ease your mind), and talk with your partner or labor coach about ways to relax and get past the anxious feelings. It's perfectly natural to be fearful of the unknown, but don't let fear wrest control of your labor from you.

Even if you have been through pregnancy already, you might still be anxious about baby's arrival. Perhaps you're following a different kind of labor and birth plan, or you're concerned about how your other child will react to his new sibling. Again, talk it out with your partner, ask your provider any questions that are still on your mind about labor and delivery, and remember that you've been through this once and you'll make it through again.

Excited and Happy

How could you not be excited? You're finally going to meet the little one you've known only through kicks, hiccups, and grainy ultrasound images. Will she look like you? What will you do when you get to hold her for the first time? Relish these final days of exhilaration and anticipation; they are unique.

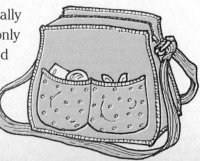

Gearing Up for the Big Event

Since baby's timetable is somewhat unpredictable, start getting your affairs in order at the beginning of this month. Cover all personal, professional, and family bases to ensure a smooth transition from home to hospital and back home again.

Finalize the Birth Plan

Double-check with your provider that a copy of your birth plan has been put into your chart, and verify any changes you might have made to the plan since your first review together. Provide your labor coach with an extra copy just in case the original is misplaced.

Pack Your Bag

You'll probably pack and unpack your bag a half dozen times this month making sure you have everything you could possibly need. Don't go crazy with books, notebook computers, or other work or entertainment equipment. You'll be too busy with labor, delivery, and the blissful preoccupation of meeting and caring for your child.

Essentials you should have:

✓ **Pain-relief tools for labor.** Things like massage balls, a picture for focusing on through contractions, a water bottle.

✓ **Music to labor by.** Check with your hospital or birthing center in advance to see whether a small portable stereo is acceptable. If not, you can always bring personal headphones.

✓ **Snacks for the coach.** Make sure it's something that won't turn your stomach if you see or smell it during labor.

✓ **A camera.** For capturing baby's arrival (or the moments shortly thereafter). Don't forget the batteries and film (or an extra memory card)!

✓ **Stopwatch, clock, or watch with a second hand.** For timing contractions.

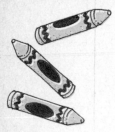

✓ **Several nightgowns.** With button or snap fronts if you're going to nurse.

✓ **Extra underwear.** Make them comfortable but not your best—they'll probably end up with some postpartum bloodstains.

✓ **Sanitary pads.** The hospital will provide you with some, but extras are good to have on hand.

✓ **Phone numbers.** Make sure your partner has names and numbers of the folks you'll want to clue in immediately on the new arrival.

✓ **A small gift from baby to any siblings.** A "hello big sister/brother" gift can make the introduction smoother.

✓ **A picture of the kids.** Taping a picture of big brother or sister to your newborn's bassinet is a good way to emphasize your first child's important new role in the family.

✓ **Glasses or contacts.** Make sure you can see the baby after he's finally here.

✓ **Warm socks and/or slippers.** Those hospital floors can be cold.

✓ **A bathrobe.** For hallway walks to the nursery.

✓ **A baby blanket.** For baby's return home. Let your partner bring the car seat on discharge day so that you aren't overwhelmed with luggage.

✓ **Toiletries.** Toothbrush, toothpaste, and other basics.

✓ **Shower supplies.** You'll be given an opportunity to shower at the hospital, so pack shampoo and other necessities.

✓ **A going-home outfit for both you and baby.** Pack a set of newborn clothes, and make sure you bring something loose and comfortable to wear yourself.

If you're breastfeeding, you might also pack:

✓ **Nursing bras.** If you don't have any yet, a bra with a front fastener will work well as a stand-in for now.

✓ **A box of nursing pads.** For when your milk comes in.

✓ **Vitamin E oil or lanolin ointment.** For sore or cracked nipples.

Recruit Help Now!

Now is the time to take friends, family, and neighbors up on their offers of assistance.

If they ask whether they can help, by all means take them up on it. Make a list and schedule assignments. Give friends who are good in the kitchen the cooking detail so that you can have a supply of frozen, home-cooked meals on hand for easy dinners. If you have other children, charge your husband or partner with making sure their school, extracurricular, and social schedules are covered.

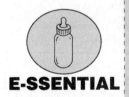

E-SSENTIAL

Don't put your prepregnancy jeans in your hospital bag. While you'll lose a large percentage of pregnancy weight at birth, it will take some time to return to your old shape and size. If the thought of yet again putting on maternity clothes postpartum is too depressing, buy a comfortable but stretchy coming-home outfit in a new-mom-friendly size.

Feel like you need some live-in help to get you through the first week or so? Ask a mommy expert, maybe even your own mom, to come for a visit. Sound out the idea with your mate; though he may feel this is a special "just the three of you" family time, he might reconsider if he hears your reasons. Just make sure your guest isn't someone who will be driving you bonkers after 2 days.

Finalize Maternity-Leave Plans

If you're working right up until your due date, start clearing the decks early in the month. Make sure coworkers and managers are regularly apprised of where outstanding projects stand, and try to treat every day as if it might be your last before you leave. The more you enable matters to flow smoothly in your absence, the less likely you are to get calls at home.

E-ALERT!

Having a cesarean section? You'll be recovering from major surgery as well as going through new-mom adjustments. It's essential that you have adequate rest and support so that you can heal and care for baby. Federal law mandates that health insurers cover at least 4 days of hospitalization following an uncomplicated C-section birth. Stay as long as you can.

Talk with your supervisor about communication during your absence. If you want to remain incommunicado (and you have every right to do so), make your feelings known. You might think about setting a limit on any contact you do agree to, such as e-mails only, which may be easier to answer at your leisure when baby is asleep, or phone calls only in a certain window of time each day. Be sure to outline circumstances that you would consider important enough to be disturbed for. Remember—this is your time off, both to recuperate and to get to know your child. Your workplace will survive.

Hurry Up and Wait (When Baby Is Late)

You've finally reached that magic EDD number and . . . nothing. No fanfare, no contractions, and definitely no baby. Disappointed, you resign yourself to yet another day of pregnancy. Don't be too depressed. Instead try to stay busy, and if you feel up to it, get out and about. A nice long walk may be just what your little one needs for inspiration. Sitting at home, analyzing every twitch of your abdomen, and watching the hours crawl by will only make the waiting longer.

Unless you have a precise 28-day cycle and are positive of the exact day that sperm met egg, gestational dating can be fuzzy at best. If you are a week or more past the EDD, your provider will order additional tests, including a biophysical profile, which includes a nonstress test and ultrasound assessment of amniotic fluid levels and fetal activity. These tools will give her a much better picture of whether or not baby is ready to arrive.

Babies who stay in the womb 42 weeks or longer are considered postdate. Postdate pregnancies can develop macrosomia, or large body size of 4,000 grams (8 pounds 13 ounces) or more that could make it difficult to pass through the birth canal. A postdate fetus may also pass meconium, the black tarry stool that is baby's first bowel movement. If meconium is released into the amniotic fluid, it has the potential to cause lung problems after the baby is born. It may also be a sign of current or past fetal distress. Postdate pregnancies are also associated with an increased risk of stillbirth and placental insufficiency (when the placenta can no longer provide enough oxygen and nutrients to the baby). That's why regular assessment of a postdate pregnancy is extremely important.

E-QUESTION

I'm a week overdue. Will my doctor induce me?
Your provider will consider several factors. Is the cervix effaced or dilated? Are you fairly sure your due date was accurate to begin with? Have you had a previous C-section? Generally speaking, if you've hit the week 41 mark and your provider thinks induction is indicated, she may broach the subject with you.

Just for Dads

It's showtime! Finally, you'll be able to get into the parenting act on a more hands-on level. As the baby's due date approaches, remember that your partner needs you more than ever. Spoil her a little—or even a lot.

Getting Her to the Hospital

Having nightmares about delivering the baby in the back seat of your Ford Taurus? Perhaps it will ease your mind to hear that the average first-time mom is in labor for about 14 hours, more than enough time to get to the hospital. (Women in second-or-beyond pregnancies tend to have shorter labors—around eight hours on average.)

Remembering everything in the thrill of the big moment may be hard, so make yourself a checklist: one overnight bag, your list of phone numbers, plenty of change or a calling card for phone calls, and—of course—one laboring mommy-to-be. And make a habit of topping off your tank every time it reaches the half-empty mark so that you won't have to stop for gas.

Many hospitals do not allow cell phone use inside the buildings due to the risk of interference with sensitive medical equipment. Although some facilities are starting to allow less obtrusive digital wireless, chances are you'll have to rely on the pay phone for now.

False Alarms

Many women hit the hospital certain that they're just hours away from birth, only to be told they're just a few centimeters dilated. There is no bigger letdown for a very pregnant woman, particularly one who is past her due date, than to be sent home from the hospital with baby still on board. She may get teary, frustrated, exasperated, and convinced that she'll be pregnant forever. Even though you, too, may be disappointed by the delay, give her a good shoulder to cry on and offer some extra TLC.

Running Interference

Taking over phone duty this month can help ease your partner's stress significantly. Chances are family, friends, neighbors, and anyone else who knows the big day is approaching will be calling for a status report. As the due date draws near, this can be a nuisance, but when the date has come and gone, it escalates into the unbearable zone. Let your spouse know you'll field the phone calls for now and pass along anything of consequence.

Labor and Delivery

Even if you've read everything ever written about labor and delivery, taken copious notes in childbirth class, watched hours of birth stories on cable TV, and questioned all your friends on their birth experiences, you'll still find your labor is different in some way from that of others. Because every woman's labor is unique, comparisons of length, progress, and pain perception can be inaccurate and even discouraging. Follow your own path, and you'll do fine.

Get Ready: Baby and Your Body in Labor

Labor is hard work (don't let anyone tell you otherwise), but it's also the most rewarding work you'll ever do.

Contractions

The first signal of labor is contractions—the tightening and release of your uterus that helps propel your baby down the birth canal. These contractions are different from the Braxton-Hicks ones you've possibly had in that they occur at regular intervals, are painful, and are slowly but surely opening the door (that is, cervix) for baby's exit.

You don't need to rush to the hospital or birthing center after your first contraction. But you should call your doctor or midwife to let her know labor has started and how far apart contractions are. Remember, contractions are timed from the beginning of one to the start of the next. Your provider will let you know at what point you should head for the hospital or birthing center. Until then, you can labor in the comfort and privacy of your own home. However, if the pain from contractions starts to be more than you can handle without professional help, have your coach call your provider back and let her know you're heading for the hospital early. Read on for early pain relief options you can try at home.

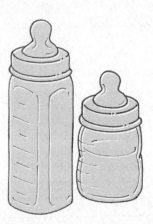

Prep

When you do arrive at your birthing center or hospital, the nursing staff will prep (prepare) you for labor and delivery. What prepping involves depends on facility policy and doctor preference, but here are some procedures you might encounter.

Suit Up

You'll change into your hospital gown or nightgown from home. Try not to wear a lot of jewelry or other extraneous items that can get lost in the shuffle from room to room.

A Close Shave

You could be getting a partial shave of your perineal area or, less commonly, a full shave of both your abdominal and pubic area.

The Enema Within

It's possible that your hospital requires an enema to clear out your bowel so that baby will have a smoother passage down the neighboring birth canal. It's not very common in today's hospitals and birth facilities, but it is a possibility. Find out in advance if this is required; you might be able to administer it at home if it makes you more comfortable. If contractions have had you on the toilet all day and you've got nothing left to give, let your nurse know and staff might bypass this step.

Drop a Line

Your nurse may insert a needle with a heparin lock and secure it to your arm with surgical tape. If intravenous (IV) medication is suddenly needed during labor, it can be easily hooked up. Other hospitals will hook you up to an IV line as a matter of course and administer a glucose solution to keep you hydrated. Other medications can be added to the line as necessary.

Baby Monitor

Chances are good that you've experienced the fetal and uterine monitors during a visit to your provider, so this part of the procedure should be familiar to you. The monitor will give you a visible and audible look at your contractions and the fetal heart rate; it will allow you and your coach to see when a contraction is coming and, more important, when it seems to be almost over. It will also pick up fetal heart sounds and alert you to any stress the baby may be experiencing from oxygen deprivation or problems with the umbilical cord. An internal monitor might be used if you are considered to be at high risk.

Get Set: Pain Relief Options

In early labor when contractions are getting intense but are still not close enough to leave for the hospital, there are a few ways you can ease the pain.

Nonmedical Solutions

First, have plenty of pillows on hand. Experiment with different positions, such as on all fours, against a wall, and leaning against someone or something while bent forward at the waist.

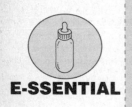

E-SSENTIAL

If you don't want to be bound to your bed during labor, find out whether your birth facility has fetal monitors that use telemetry. These wireless monitors strap on like a regular external device so that you don't have to remain plugged into anything. There are even telemetry units that are waterproof, if you plan on easing labor pains with hydrotherapy.

Back labor, which occurs when baby's face is toward your abdomen rather than toward your spine, can cause severe lower-back pain. Ask your partner to try massage or a warm water bottle to ease contractions. The soothing jets of a whirlpool tub can do wonders, if you have one. If your water has broken, however, never take a soak without approval from your provider.

Keep positive, supportive people around you. Let your coach be your buffer and clear out any distractions. Try to remain focused on riding through and past the contraction. Fix your eyes on something that relaxes you and practice the breathing exercises you learned in childbirth class to keep the oxygen and blood flowing. Don't hyperventilate. Talk or groan through the peak of the contraction if it helps.

It's difficult to relax while you're in the midst of a really big, really uncomfortable contraction. However, letting go in between contractions can help ease your mind and body and loosen you up for impending delivery. You probably learned a few relaxation exercises in childbirth class. If so, now is the time to try them, as they can make the pain more manageable.

Progressive relaxation, a series of muscle tightening and releasing, is a good way to release your stress. Make sure you're in comfortable clothes in a soothing atmosphere (that is, quiet and perhaps dim). Recline with your head and back elevated, then start tensing and releasing each muscle group, from your head to your toes. Breathe in with the tension, and blow out with the release. Try to clear your head of everything but the sensation at hand. If you practice this prior to labor, it can be a good tool for managing some of the early pain when contractions are still relatively far apart.

Pharmaceutical Options

Once you arrive at the hospital, you will have analgesics and anesthetics available for pain relief, if you choose to use them.

Analgesics

Analgesics deaden the pain by depressing your nervous system. They make you sleepy and help you rest between contractions. The analgesics Demerol (meperidine), Stadol (butorphanol), Nubain (nalbuphine), and Sublimaze (fentanyl) are commonly used in labor. Although some of these drugs, such as Demerol, can even allow you to nap between contractions, you remain conscious under their influence (albeit a bit giddy). Although these medications can cross the placenta, when they are properly administered in the appropriate dosages they should not cause baby any serious side effects.

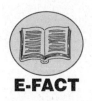

E-FACT

Pain relief in labor was roundly condemned for many centuries, partly on biblical grounds (think Eve and the apple), until Queen Victoria of England requested and was administered chloroform for the birth of her eighth and ninth children. The resultant births of Prince Leopold and Princess Beatrice were attended by a pioneer in anesthetic use, Dr. John Snow.

General Anesthesia

You may also receive either a general or local (regional) anesthetic. General anesthesia brings about a complete loss of consciousness ("puts you to sleep"). General anesthesia is rarely used in labor and delivery, usually only in cases of an emergency cesarean section when there isn't adequate time to prep the patient with a local anesthetic. Newborns arriving under the influence of a general anesthesia can be drowsy and slow to respond due to the effects of the anesthesia.

Local Anesthesia

Local anesthesia, also called *regional anesthesia*, numbs only a specific portion of the body and leaves you awake and alert. The most commonly used local anesthesia is probably the lumbar epidural. Injected into the space between two vertebrae of your lower back (in the epidural space), this type of anesthesia is administered when you are well into labor; it will temporarily numb the nerves all the way from your bellybutton to your knees. An epidural takes 20 minutes to start working and can lower your blood pressure, so you'll be put on the fetal monitor and hooked up to an IV fluid drip if you're given an epidural.

Some providers may require you to wait until you reach a certain dilation benchmark or stage of labor to have an epidural. But if you are being induced, an epidural might be in order earlier because you can experience a lot of pain before there is any major progress in the dilation of your cervix. With an epidural most providers will give you more time to push because your sensation is impaired. If you have concerns about epidural timing, discuss them with your health care provider.

The epidural is administered through a small plastic catheter in your back. An anesthesiologist will place the epidural catheter and administer the local anesthetic agent. Before he starts, your lower back will be draped and the insertion spot swabbed with antiseptic or iodine. You might be asked to pull your knees and chin toward your chest so that your spine is more visible. The catheter is inserted in the space between the fourth and fifth vertebrae, and the anesthesia injected. You may feel a slight stinging sensation

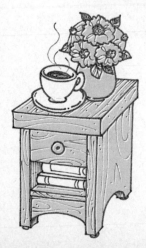

down your legs, but your breathing and the involuntary muscles working those contractions won't be affected. The insertion of an epidural catheter allows anesthetics to be administered on an as-needed basis and is useful should a C-section be required.

When insertion is complete, the doctor will secure the catheter and you can get comfortable again. Watch the fetal monitor for the start of the next contraction. You'll be amazed at how what was turning you inside out a moment ago is barely perceptible now. The numbness will take several hours to wear off and may restrict your movements during the birth, but an epidural can be a great pain management tool.

A spinal block is similar to an epidural in that it's administered in the lower back. However, a spinal is delivered directly into your lower spine, not into the spaces between your vertebrae as in an epidural. Used right at delivery only or during a C-section, the spinal will numb you from your rib cage all the way down.

Women who want the pain relief benefits of an epidural but also wish to retain the ability to move around during labor are candidates for a low-dose combination spinal epidural, sometimes referred to as a *walking epidural*. An epidural catheter is inserted, and an injection of a narcotic is administered into the spinal fluid using a smaller needle that fits through the epidural catheter. A walking epidural is usually faster acting than a conventional epidural and allows you to retain enough sensation to move and walk, which can speed the labor process.

Other anesthetic blocks that are used less frequently include:

- **A caudal block** is administered into the bony area right at the end of your spine; it affects the abdominal and pelvic muscles.
- **A saddle block** is a type of low spinal anesthesia that numbs a more limited area of your body—your perineum, inner thighs, and buttocks.
- **With a paracervical block,** the anesthetic is injected into either side of your cervix during labor to numb the area.
- **With a pudendal block,** the anesthetic is administered to the nerves around the vagina and pelvic floor to help control pain when the baby's head bulges into your cervix.

Go! Labor in Three Acts

Labor is a series of three distinct stages, aptly called *first*, *second*, and *third stages*. For most women the longest span is the first stage, which lasts from the earliest signs of labor right through baby's descent into the birth canal, in preparation for stage two—pushing. Stage three consists of delivering the placenta; mothers usually feel this is a cakewalk after all the hard work involved in baby's arrival.

First Stage

The first stage of labor begins with early (latent) labor and ends with active labor. Your provider probably uses the term transition (descent) to refer to the end of first-stage labor.

During the early phase the cervix effaces (thins) and dilates (opens). This ripening process perhaps started several weeks ago, well before the regular contractions of early labor began. Now your cervix will dilate to about 4 or 5 centimeters. Contractions will arrive every 15 to 20 minutes and last 60 to 90 seconds. If your partner or coach isn't around, now is the time to contact him so that he can be by your side. Then touch bases with your provider, who will tell you at what point you should head to the hospital or birthing facility.

Try to stay up and moving through contractions as much as you can to let gravity help your baby descend. Consider a light liquid snack (for example, broth or juice) to power up your energy reserves for the long road ahead. Rest if possible. Try the breathing and relaxation techniques you picked up in childbirth class as well as the coach-assisted massage or showering to get you through these first few hours. Then leave for the hospital and the next phase—active labor.

In active labor your contractions are coming closer together regularly, perhaps 3 to 5 minutes apart, and they can be intense, lasting 45 to 60 seconds. These strong contractions are dilating your cervix from about 4 or 5 centimeters to around 8.

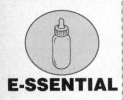

E-SSENTIAL

If your birthing center or hospital has whirlpool tubs or showers available for laboring moms, you might find the pulsating water welcome relief for getting through contractions. This pain relief method (called *hydrotherapy*) is not the same as a water birth, in which a baby is actually born submerged in a pool of water.

Once you reach the birthing center or hospital, you'll be quickly prepped as described earlier and given an internal exam to check the dilation of your cervix. The baby's position will be checked, and you will probably be hooked up to a fetal monitor to assess the baby's well-being.

Other signs that active labor is in progress:

✓ **Your membranes rupture.** If the amniotic sac hasn't already broken, it will now or very soon.

✓ **You bleed from your vagina.** More of the mucous plug is being expelled.

✓ **You need air.** Put those cleansing breaths and other breathing techniques into practice. Your hard-working uterus needs oxygen.

✓ **Your back really hurts.** The baby's head is pushing on your backbone. Massage can help.

✓ **You have muscle cramps.** Again, massage can help the ill-timed charley horse.

✓ **You're exhausted and physically spent.** Remember what you're working toward. Let your coach know how you're feeling so that she can motivate you and get you whatever she can to keep you moving forward.

Don't feel inadequate or guilty about asking for pain medication at any point if you want it. You wouldn't hesitate to take Novocain if you were getting a wisdom tooth pulled, yet having an 8-pound child pulled through a 10-centimeter opening doesn't qualify? Pain medication is a tool, just like your breathing exercises. Wisely used, it can result in a better birth experience for both you and your child.

Once your cervix reaches 8 centimeters and contractions start coming one on top of another to get you to full dilation, the end of the first stage (transition) has arrived. Because of the frequency of contractions and the overwhelming urge to push, this is the most difficult part of labor. Fortunately, it culminates in your child's delivery, once you bridge those final 2 centimeters to become fully dilated.

As you begin to transition from first- to second-stage labor:

✓ You can become nauseated and may even vomit.

✓ You have chills or sweats, and your muscles twitch.

✓ Your back *really, really* hurts.

✓ Contractions are just minutes apart, if even that.

✓ There is pressure in your rectum from the baby.

✓ You are absolutely exhausted.

✓ You may feel like pushing even though your cervix is not yet fully dilated.

Although every fiber of your body is probably screaming "PUSH!," you need to hold back just a few moments more. Your cervix is almost, but not quite, open far enough for baby's safe passage. Take quick, shallow breaths and resist the urge to push until your doctor or midwife gives the go-ahead.

Second Stage, or PUSH!

Your cervix has made it to 10 centimeters, and you are finally allowed to push. This second stage can last anywhere from a few minutes (with second or subsequent babies) to several hours. Your contractions will still arrive regularly, but they aren't quite as close together—a welcome relief. Pushing is very hard work, but the sensations may change from the intense gripping you've experienced to more of a stinging or burning sensation.

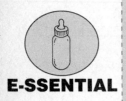

E-SSENTIAL

If possible, try to find a pushing position that makes you feel comfortable and in control. Use gravity to your advantage by kneeling, squatting, or sitting up with your legs and knees spread far apart. Stirrups are likely available, but don't feel forced into using them if they don't work for you.

Your birth attendant and/or coach will let you know when the peak of the contraction occurs, the optimum time for pushing effectively. Use whatever it takes to push effectively. If that means moaning, grunting, and emitting other primal sounds that make your prenatal snoring sound like a lullaby by comparison, go for it. The people attending your birth have probably heard just about everything. Don't be embarrassed, because the noise won't even faze them.

The emergence of the head at your vaginal opening starts with a small patch of skin visible during the peak of a push. The patch may recede when you rest but will reappear at the next contraction. Unless your baby is arriving in a breech position, the head will finally crown (bulge) right out of your vaginal opening. You may be asked to stop pushing momentarily as the baby's head is ready to emerge, in order to prevent perineal tearing. Panting can help you suppress the urge. The obstetrician or midwife may decide on an episiotomy if your skin doesn't appear willing to stretch another millimeter, or she may attempt perineal massage.

Finally the head slides face down past the perineum and is eased out carefully by the birth attendant to prevent injury to the baby. The attendant may wipe the eyes, nose, and mouth and suction any mucus or fluid from her upper respiratory tract. It's all downhill from here as the rest of the body slides out.

As your baby leaves the quiet, dim warmth of the womb for the bright lights and big noises of the outside world, his respiratory reflexes kick in and the newborn lungs fill with air for the first time. He'll probably test out those lungs with a full-fledged wail. Your doctor will place the baby on your stomach for introductions, usually with the umbilical cord still attached.

The cord will continue to pulse with blood flow for a few minutes. The timing of the actual clamping and severing of the cord will depend upon your practitioner, and this is a matter of some debate in childbirth circles. Some professionals believe that waiting until pulsation has stopped or even until after the placenta is delivered improves baby's circulation and blood pressure, reducing baby's risk of early childhood anemia and mom's chance of hemorrhage. Other practitioners still follow the traditional method of clamping and cutting the cord earlier. You may want to talk the issue over with your doctor in advance of delivery day if you have concerns about the timing of the cord cut. If baby requires resuscitation, or if the cord is tightly wrapped around a body part or is exceedingly short, it will be cut sooner.

Most practitioners will give dad (or even mom) the option of cutting the cord in an uncomplicated birth. Don't feel bad if it isn't your cup of tea, especially if either one of you is a bit squeamish. Better to spend the time cuddling your baby than being picked up off the delivery room floor.

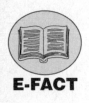

E-FACT

A 2006 Cochrane Review found that delayed clamping of the umbilical cord for preterm infants may improve health outcomes. Among preemies who had a delay in cord clamping of anywhere from 30 seconds to 2 minutes, the risk of intraventricular hemorrhage (bleeding on the brain) and the need for postpartum transfusion were significantly reduced.

Some parents choose to bank their child's umbilical cord blood and/ or placenta blood after birth. This blood contains stem cells, those miraculous little blank slates from which all organs and tissues are built. Cord and/ or placenta blood collected immediately after birth is placed in a collection kit and flown to a facility where it is cryogenically frozen and banked for later use, if needed. The theory behind banking this at birth is that if your child ever develops a disease or condition requiring stem-cell treatment, the blood can be thawed and used for her treatment. If it matches certain biological markers, it may be used to treat other family members as well. However, banking is cost prohibitive for many and requires an ongoing annual storage fee.

Third Stage, or You Aren't Done Yet!

The third stage of labor is the delivery of the placenta. The entire placenta must be expelled to prevent bleeding and infection complications later on. Contractions will continue, and your doctor may press down on your abdomen and massage your uterus or tug gently on the end of the umbilical cord hanging from your vagina. You might also be injected with the hormone Pitocin (oxytocin) to step up your contractions and expel the placenta. You'll be given pushing directives again, but this part will seem like a piece of cake given the task you've just completed.

Once the placenta is out, any stitches you require to repair tearing or episiotomy incisions will be put in. A local anesthetic will be injected to deaden the area if you aren't still anesthetized from an epidural.

Cesarean Section

A cesarean birth will be scheduled for you if you have a breech baby or other complications or conditions that indicate the need for such. It may also be performed in emergency situations in which the fetus is in distress. A cesarean is major abdominal surgery and carries with it all the risks of infection and complication that any surgical procedure does. On the positive side, with a planned C-section, the date your physician schedules the procedure is your due date, and no contractions are necessary unless you begin to labor before that time.

In Advance of the Surgery

If you have any advance warning about your C-section, you'll probably be offered an epidural or spinal rather than general anesthesia. Before the procedure begins, you'll be prepped. A nurse may shave the area of the incision, and your arm will be hooked up to an intravenous line to receive fluids as well as pain medication. You may also be asked to drink an antacid solution called *sodium citrate* to neutralize your stomach acid.

E-ALERT!

If you are having a scheduled cesarean, try to arrange a few moments to consult with the anesthesiologist ahead of time. If you've had any poor experiences with anesthesia in prior C-sections, let her know so that you can improve the outcome this time around. She can also answer any questions you might have about her part of the procedure.

Before the procedure begins, you will have a catheter inserted into your bladder. The anesthetic block will give you little control over the muscles that control urine flow, so the catheter will do the work for you, both during and after the procedure. Catheter insertion can be uncomfortable, so ask that it be inserted after you've received your anesthetic block (which will likely be in the operating room).

In the Operating Room

Once you're prepped, you will be wheeled to the operating room. In the operating room, the anesthesiologist will have you roll on your side and pull your knees toward your chest (or sit on the edge of the table with your legs hanging off) while he inserts a fine needle and catheter for an epidural or spinal block into your back. You'll then be asked to lie flat on your back with your arms straight out to the sides. A curtain just a few feet high will be positioned at your chest to keep the surgical field (the area where all the action is) sterile. This will also block your view of the procedure, so if you're determined to see baby the moment she emerges, you will want to ask for an appropriately placed mirror as early as possible.

Your arms may be loosely fastened down with Velcro straps. This is not to keep you from jumping off the table but to prevent any accidental movements that could breech the sterility of the surgical field.

The most uncomfortable part of the C-section procedure is arguably the flat-on-your-back part. It's quite possible you will become nauseated as your heavy uterus compresses your vena cava and starts to lower your blood pressure. In addition, the anesthetic itself may cause your blood pressure to fall. Although the anesthesiologist will administer medication to control this drop (called *hypotension*) you may get sick to your stomach. Think how long you can tolerate lying flat on your back at 9-months pregnant, and you'll see why. The discomfort is compounded by the fact that you will have to vomit lying down with your head turned to the side. This is where a well-placed mate, tray in hand, is indispensable. If this does happen, hang in there and remember this part will likely be short-lived.

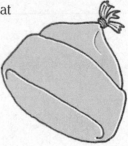

A postdural puncture headache or spinal headache is a potential side effect of spinal blocks and epidurals. It's caused by the change in spinal fluid pressure that occurs if fluid leaks out into the epidural space following the procedure. When rest and fluids don't help, an injection of blood into the epidural space (a blood patch) may be required to ease the pain.

The obstetrician will make an incision, and the baby's head, perfectly round because she hasn't done battle with the birth canal, will be lifted out first and her mouth and nose suctioned. As your doctor helps your baby out of the incision, you'll feel a strange pulling sensation. Once the cord is cut, you'll be able to finally see your baby, albeit briefly, before she is taken for assessment and a quick cleanup by the nursing staff. In some cases the pediatric team will be in the operating room to assess the baby immediately. Your incision will be stitched closed, and you'll be wheeled off to the recovery room where your little one will meet up with you once again. The entire surgical procedure will only take about 30 to 45 minutes.

Emergency C-Section

If your C-section is performed under emergency circumstances, events could move quickly and you'll have fewer options. You could also be given a general anesthetic that will make you unconscious. Most dads are asked to step outside once general anesthesia has been administered, but you might want to talk to your doctor about special circumstances during childbirth.

Induction

In cases in which you are at term and it seems your child is perfectly content to spend his infancy in your womb, your practitioner may recommend induction. Before induction, your provider will verify that the gestational age of your baby is at least 39 weeks by using ultrasound, Doppler, and pregnancy test records.

Inducing labor involves both helping the cervix ripen for baby's passage and stimulating uterine contractions; both are important for a successful labor and delivery. If the cervix is not adequately effaced and dilated, the chance of interventions (for example, C-section or use of forceps) goes up. If you are a first-time mom, you are at increased risk of having a cesarean section as a result of a "failed induction."

Cervical ripening decreases the chance of failed induction. Your provider may use one of several methods to facilitate cervical ripening, including membrane stripping and amniotomy (manual breaking of the membranes or bag of waters). Stripping (sweeping) of the membranes is simply the separation of the amniotic membrane from the wall of the cervix. Your provider will insert her finger in the cervix and gently sweep it between the amniotic membrane and the uterine wall.

If she opts for amniotomy, she'll use an instrument with a small blunt hook on the end (an amnihook) to break through the amniotic sac. With the latter method, if labor does not start on its own within 24 hours, scheduled induction may be necessary because of the risk of infection for the baby.

E-ALERT!

Amniotic fluid that is greenish or brown in color may contain meconium, your baby's first bowel movement. The presence of meconium can indicate fetal distress. If you are leaking amniotic fluid and there are signs of meconium, the situation should be evaluated by your provider immediately.

Because a scheduled induction is more successful when the cervix is prepared for the experience, your practitioner may recommend an application of prostaglandin to your cervix the day prior or in the hospital. The prostaglandin helps to ripen the cervix for labor and delivery. In some cases it can be used alone as an inducing agent. The prostaglandin can take the form of a gel or tablet and can be inserted into the vagina. On some occasions the tablet is given orally. The baby's heart rate is assessed with a fetal monitor after the prostaglandin is given and during labor. More than one application may be ordered.

Manual dilators and Foley catheters can also be used for cervical ripening, as an alternative to the use of drugs. The type of cervical ripening method used depends on your personal preference, your medical history, and the cervical exam. Prostaglandins are not used in induction in women with a previous cesarean section because they can increase the risk of uterine rupture.

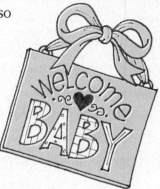

Pitocin, a synthetic formulation of the hormone oxytocin that stimulates uterine contractions, may be prescribed as an inducing agent. The hormone is given intravenously, and you will be hooked up to a fetal monitor to monitor your baby's progress.

The rate of labor induction in the United States has more than doubled over the past decade. Researchers attribute the increase to earlier prenatal care, wider availability of induction agents, and nonmedical reasons such as convenience for the patient or doctor. Because induction can cause intense contractions and result in a longer labor, its use should always be carefully considered.

After the Birth

The pinnacle of 9 months of physical chaos and emotional oscillation, of queasy stomach, lost car keys, aches, pains, and hair-trigger laughter and tears, has arrived. Your baby is here, placed skin to skin to feel his mother's outside warmth for the very first time.

Meeting Baby

A thousand different feelings and emotions, from utter exhaustion to indescribable joy, will flood you as you look down at that little scrunched face, still adjusting to his new waterless environment. Wrapped in a blanket with a little stocking cap to keep his head warm, he looks so perfect yet so vulnerable.

If you're planning on breastfeeding, you can nurse him while you get acquainted, even in the recovery room if you've had a C-section. It's awe inspiring how he knows just what to do, instinctively rooting for your breast with his eyes barely open and then latching on. Spend as long as you want getting familiar, and let baby's daddy share in the bonding, too. This is a precious time for your new family.

Baby's First Doctor Visit

After you've met your child, she'll need some initial tests and treatments to ensure a healthy welcome into the world. The first is an Apgar test, which is simply an assessment of baby's reactivity, health, and appearance at birth. Created by noted pediatrician Dr. Virginia Apgar, the Apgar measures Appearance (skin color), Pulse, Grimace (reflexes), Activity, and Respiration. The Apgar is given just 1 minute after birth and again 5 minutes after that. The attendant will assign a score of 0 to 2 for each category and add the numbers together for the total Apgar. An average score is 7 to 10.

After the Apgar, your newborn will be measured, weighed, and have prints taken of her feet and fingers. Silver nitrate or antibiotic eye drops or ointment may be put in her eyes to prevent infection from anything she encountered in the birth canal. She'll also receive a vitamin K injection to prevent bleeding problems and a heel-stick blood draw to test for phenylketonuria (PKU), hypothyroidism, and a variety of other medical issues (screenings vary by the state your child is born in). Further tests may be administered if you have a chronic illness or have experienced complications during pregnancy. If you have diabetes, for example, your newborn will have her blood glucose (sugar) levels tested. The American Academy of Pediatrics also recommends that all infants get a hearing test and receive a hepatitis B vaccine before leaving the hospital.

Taking Care of Mom

After the birth you'll have some assistance cleaning up and will be given a good supply of super-absorbent sanitary pads. You'll also be provided with a peri bottle, a plastic squirt bottle used to cleanse and soothe your perineal area with warm water each time you use the bathroom.

You'll be expelling lochia for up to 6 weeks following birth, whether you've had a vaginal birth or a C-section. Lochia—a mixture of blood, mucus, and tissue that comes from the implantation site of the placenta—

will be quite heavy in the days immediately following the birth, so don't be alarmed.

If bleeding is soaking more than a pad an hour, let your provider know. It could be a sign that a piece of placenta is still retained in your uterus. This condition usually requires surgical removal of the placental fragments, a procedure called *curettage*.

If you've had a C-section, you'll spend some time in the recovery area before heading to your hospital room. Your incision will be checked regularly, and pain medication will be administered as needed. The next day you'll be encouraged to walk as soon as possible to get your digestive tract active again, and you'll be asked about your gas and bathroom habits ad nauseum. The nursing staff is just trying to ensure that everything is returning to normal in gastrointestinal land.

Women who are given episiotomies will take sitz baths (also known as *hip baths*) to relieve pain, promote healing, and keep the area clean. A sitz bath is a small, shallow tub of water, sometimes with medication added, that you sit in. Some mild pain relievers may also be prescribed to ease episiotomy pain.

Hospital Stay

Many hospitals have rooming in, in which your baby can sleep in your hospital room with you and you can begin the process of learning to care for and comfort him. It's a marvelous way to promote early bonding. However, if you are exhausted and your little guy seems to be having a problem getting to sleep, don't hesitate to get some help from the nursing staff. If you need a nap, they can wheel him down to the nursery for a few hours while you sleep. Childbirth, whether vaginally or by C-section, takes a physical toll from which you need to recover in order to parent effectively.

For the same reason, don't feel bad about keeping visitors to a minimum. Your hospital will have a visitor's policy, which will help somewhat. Although introducing immediate family members to their new relative is important, friends, neighbors, and coworkers can wait. At many facilities, you can also request that the switchboard hold phone calls to your room. Anyone who has a cold or other infection, even a family member, should not come in contact with your baby right now because of the risk of infection, and hand washing is a must for all visitors. Your baby's little immune system is just starting to rev up.

E-ALERT!

> Recovery from a C-section will take a bit longer than from a vaginal delivery. When you laugh, sneeze, or cough, hold onto your incision with both hands. You'll find that using extra pillows for support over the incision area will allow you to cuddle and breastfeed your baby in comfort.

If you are planning on breastfeeding, now is the perfect time to get your technique down. Your OB nurses will likely ask you how breastfeeding is progressing, and they may request that you write down the time and frequency of nursing so that they can assess baby's progress. They can also examine your latching technique to help you troubleshoot if breastfeeding isn't yet going smoothly. In some cases there is even a lactation consultant available, and hospitals frequently offer breastfeeding classes to their new-mother inpatients.

Remember that even though it will take a few days for your breasts to start manufacturing milk, you are already providing your child with nutrient-rich colostrum, the prelude to breastmilk. When your milk does arrive (come in), about the third day after delivery, your breasts can be quite swollen, hard, and sore. This engorgement will be relieved upon nursing.

If you're going the bottle route, cold packs and supportive bras or binding can ease the discomfort. The tenderness of engorgement usually passes in 2 to 3 days and can be relieved by mild analgesics as prescribed by your doctor. While you wait for your milk supply to dry up again (usually a period of about 2 weeks), you can use nursing pads to prevent leaks.

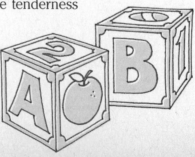

On Your Mind

Mortified by the possibility of losing control—both physically and emotionally —during labor? Childbirth is hard, painful work, and you need to work through it in your own way. The people around you are medical professionals and know this. Pain—in addition to the ultimate goal of meeting your child—is a great motivator for getting past feelings of fear or bashfulness.

Many women who were previously shy or self-conscious about their bodies find that pregnancy and motherhood pretty much eradicate any lingering traces of modesty. When you're in labor, you don't care if the attending doctor is animal, vegetable, or mineral; your mind and body are entirely focused on the impending arrival of your child. After they've been through the birth experience, many women find that there's virtually nothing that can embarrass them.

E-QUESTION

Should we have our son circumcised?
The American Academy of Pediatrics states that there are currently no firm medical or hygienic grounds for performing routine circumcision in newborn boys. However, they also cite the importance of weighing cultural and religious beliefs and the child's best interest in the decision to circumcise or not. If circumcision is performed, the AAP recommends analgesic pain relief for the infant.

Just for Dads

Until today, your most important function seemed to have been back rubs and the Saturday night cheesecake run. But as labor starts, you will see just how pivotal your presence is in the childbirth process.

Coaching Your Team

You'll wear a number of hats as coach—gopher, massage therapist, hall monitor, motivational speaker, and advocate. Your partner must focus completely on the task at hand, and she will rely on your support for quashing distractions and attending to her needs.

Don't be offended if you're told to take your stopwatch and cram it, or if she impatiently shoos you away as you try to regulate her breathing. She still wants you and, more important, needs you by her side. Be flexible, stick with it, and work with her toward your common goal of a beautiful, healthy baby.

Reassurance for the Faint of Heart

Birth, both by C-section and vaginally, can be a very blood-soaked scene. Chances are the rush of seeing your baby emerge will overwhelm any aversions to blood and other bodily fluids. But if it doesn't, don't feel bad about taking a moment to collect yourself—outside the delivery room if need be. A nurse or another support person can stand in for you in the meantime. Now is not the time to faint, fall, and get a concussion (although many an expectant dad has passed out in the heat of the moment). One tip—if you are known for getting the whim-whams at the sight of blood, you and your partner should discuss the possibility of your early exit before labor. You might want to have a stand-by coach just in case.

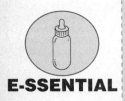

E-SSENTIAL

If your partner is having a C-section, there will be a surgical curtain or drape positioned above her belly. Typically dad is positioned by mom's head for emotional support throughout the procedure. To avoid the sight of blood and of your significant other's internal organs, stay below the sight line of the surgical drape by remaining seated on a stool by your partner's head.

The Best Laid Plans

Things can go wrong in childbirth, but the more you know about complications in advance, the easier it is to deal with them should they arise.

Emergency Birth

In cases in which the fetus begins to show signs of distress (rapid acceleration or sudden slowdown of fetal heart rate) or you experience a life-threatening condition such as hemorrhage, you will be rushed to the OR for an emergency cesarean. In most cases, because time is of the essence, you will be given a general anesthetic.

Women who attempt a vaginal birth after a cesarean (VBAC) can be at risk for uterine rupture or a separation of their previous C-section scar. If this occurs, an emergency C-section is performed. It should be noted, however, that the success rate of VBAC is very good: Between 60 and 80 percent of individuals who are considered candidates for the procedure come through it with flying colors.

Delivery Complications

A child with a head too large for passage through the pelvis (called *cephalopelvic disproportion*), a labor that fails to progress past 6 or 7 centimeters despite best efforts, or fetal distress caused by a compressed umbilical cord are all possible complications that could cause an unplanned cesarean section.

In cases in which your baby needs a little extra help getting out of the birth canal, the use of forceps may be required. This tong-like device is used to reach into the birth canal, gently grasp the baby's head, and pull him out. Forceps are also used to reposition a baby who is intent on arriving in a poor position. The terms mid- and low-forceps delivery indicate where the doctor inserts the instrument into the birth canal. When forceps are used at all, the low position is the more likely one.

Sometimes forceps are used simply to lift the baby up and out right there at your perineum; this use is called *outlet forceps*. Babies delivered via forceps do wear signs of these instruments as bruises or red marks on either side of their heads for a few days, and there is a very slim risk of brain injury.

If your provider is concerned that using forceps will injure your perineal tissues, he may choose vacuum extraction instead. Suctioned onto the baby's head, a cup is attached to a chain or handle that the doctor pulls on while you keep on pushing. The cup will simply fall off the baby's head if too much pressure builds up. However, babies who arrive via vacuum extraction can have a bruised, swollen look on the tops of their heads.

Other maternal complications can occur following a successful delivery. Postpartum hemorrhage and a related dive in blood pressure can occur when the uterus fails to contract again after both baby and placenta have been delivered. Compression and massage of the uterus and/or drug therapy might be used to stop the bleeding. In cases in which a tear of the cervix has occurred, this will be sutured. If these measures still don't stop the bleeding, surgery may be required.

Breastfeeding Basics

Breastfeeding is one part instinct, one part practice, and a whole lot of persistence and patience. It's this last part that makes the difference between breast and bottle for many women, particularly in the first weeks of motherhood when even minor nursing difficulties can seem insurmountable. Stick with it, and take advantage of help and advice from other moms and from your health care providers. The good news is that breastfeeding usually becomes easier and more fulfilling over time.

Breast or Bottle?

Are you going to breastfeed or go the formula route? It's an issue over which many new moms feel intense pressure, and if you're still undecided you've likely heard extensive opinions on both sides of the subject. Which is the right choice?

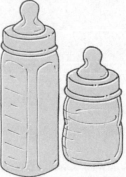

If you compare breastmilk to formula strictly on a nutrient basis, few would disagree that the better choice is breastmilk. But since the issue is also loaded with social, emotional, and personal considerations, the matter is seldom so black and white. In the end, breast or bottle is an individual choice.

Pros and Cons

A plus feature of breastfeeding for one woman is a minus for another. Consider the pros and cons of breast and bottle and how these fit with your particular life and family situation.

BREASTFEEDING PROS AND CONS:

PRO: The hands-down perfect food for your child, breastmilk is custom-made for her nutritional needs and provides her with essential antibodies.

CON: If you have a medical condition that requires drug treatment, it's possible your medication can pass into breastmilk and potentially pose a risk to baby. (Talk with your doctor if this is the case; you may have other treatment options.)

PRO: Breastfeeding is a low-maintenance feeding routine. It's always close at hand and never needs mixing, warming, or other preparation.

CON: In the beginning, at least, you will always need to be close at hand as well. Breastfeeding can be as physically taxing as it is emotionally rewarding.

PRO: Nursing gives you special one-on-one bonding time with baby.

CON: Breasts don't detach. No one else can pitch in on the feeding duties.

PRO: If you're on a budget, breastfeeding is a big cost cutter. Aside from the high cost of formula itself, you can save on bottles, bags, cleaning gadgets, and other formula-feeding purchases.

CON: You might have to purchase or rent a breast pump and buy a personal kit to use with it, and this can also be costly.

PRO: As a breastfeeding mom, you're taking part in a tradition as old as motherhood itself and giving your child something no one else can. The experience is priceless.

CON: Unfortunately, there are still many unenlightened knuckleheads out there who can't get past their perception of the breast as strictly a sexual object and who will relegate you to the corner or the closet, if given the chance.

PRO: Many women who breastfeed experience faster postpartum weight loss.

CON: Although you may be taking your figure back, your breasts belong to baby—leaks, sore nipples, and all.

BOTTLE-FEEDING PROS AND CONS:

PRO: Feeding isn't only mom, all day and all night. Your partner can get up at 4 A.M. once in a while to feed the baby.

CON: Feeding isn't only mom, all day and all night. The special mother-child bond and skin-to-skin contact that breastfeeding brings can be harder to achieve.

PRO: You can give your baby a bottle just about anywhere, anytime without feeling self-conscious or raising eyebrows.

CON: Before you hit the road, make sure you pack sterilized bottles and nipples, formula, bottled water for mixing powdered formula, and an ice pack if you've made the bottles in advance. If the bottles are chilled, you need a place to warm them, and don't forget the extra formula in case you're gone longer than you anticipated. Convenience is in the eye of the beholder.

PRO: No worries about keeping up your milk supply when you return to work.

CON: You may miss out on a golden opportunity to spend special nursing time together at home once your busy work schedule starts encroaching on family time again.

PRO: You can assume control of your body again after many months away from the helm.

CON: After so many months as one, you're suddenly severing a close physical bond that nursing can prolong.

E-QUESTION

I'm going back to work soon. Should I even bother breastfeeding now?

Even a short period of breastfeeding can have big advantages for your baby. Many women do return to work and continue to nurse. Pumping breastmilk, and gradually reducing the number of feedings to nurse in the morning and the evening only (and supplementing with formula), are options.

Being Comfortable with Your Decision

You are not an uncaring and self-absorbed mother if you choose to bottle-feed. Likewise, if you breastfeed your child openly and even through toddlerhood, you are not a militant Mother-Earth nut.

Try to weigh the risks versus the benefits in your situation. All things being equal, women who are well supported at home, are healthy, and don't face an excessively demanding work schedule should consider giving breastfeeding a try even if they feel a little awkward about it. Often the awkwardness evaporates with a little practice and through the bond forged with baby in nursing. And the health benefits gained by baby will last a lifetime.

On the other hand, if you're a single mom who works two jobs and is already stretched to the limit emotionally and physically, don't be pressured into breastfeeding by others because it is "the right thing to do." Excessive stress can do more damage than good, impairing your parenting skills, putting your health at risk, and straining the time the two of you do have together. Not every life situation is ideal for breastfeeding, even if you are capable of doing it. Make the decision that works best for your family.

Your Body and Breastfeeding

As soon as you can hold baby, you can breastfeed her. In the first few days following birth, your breasts will produce that clear-to-yellow sticky substance: *colostrum*. Colostrum contains antibodies that help strengthen the infant immune system. It also is important for getting baby's digestion off on the right track. The low-carbohydrate, high-protein concoction is easily digestible in these early days and helps to establish intestinal flora (beneficial bacteria) in baby's gastrointestinal tract. It also encourages the passing of meconium, your infant's first stools.

Colostrum comes out in small amounts compared to later breastmilk, which will fill the alveoli (sacs connected to the milk ducts) of your breasts about 3 days after birth. You'll know when your milk "comes in": Your breasts will become engorged with milk, be rock hard, and feel sore to the touch. Nursing your baby will relieve the pressure quickly, although it's possible you will need a little additional help to ease soreness. A few clinical studies have shown some benefit in the use of cabbage leaves (yes, cabbage leaves) to relieve the discomfort of engorgement. Massage and warm compresses can also help.

Latching and Letdown

Some babies seem to be breastfeeding champs from the get-go, while others need a little coaching. You're both new at this, so have patience and remember that you'll get better with practice. If you're having a hospital stay after your birth, the nurses on the maternity ward can give you some pointers on technique and check baby's latching on. In some cases there will be a lactation specialist on staff to consult with.

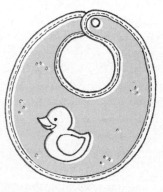

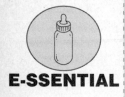

Sore or dry and cracked nipples are common phenomena as you get on the breastfeeding launch pad. Never fear: They will toughen up. In the meantime, try vitamin E oil for moisturizing, or pure lanolin ointment for easing abrasions and pain. You'll only need a tiny dollop of each, applied right after nursing. Just wipe the vitamin E oil off your nipples thoroughly before baby feeds again.

Start with a comfortable position for the two of you. Baby's whole body should face yours—not just her turned head. The cradle and cross-cradle holds are two common positions. The cradle holds your baby close across the front of your body, with her head in the crook of your arm and your hand supporting her bottom. The cross-cradle switches arms and puts your hand under her head. Lying down with baby facing you is a good choice for the utterly exhausted.

The football position (clutch hold) tucks baby under your arm, again facing your body and breast. If you've had a C-section, this can help by keeping the weight off your incision. It's also a favorite of moms with twins who are doing double nursing duty.

The seated Australian hold (in which the baby sits in your lap facing your breast) might be a good choice if you'd like to try to keep baby awake during and after his feeding. With all nursing positions, make sure your baby's head is well supported.

After you're settled into position, brace your breast with one hand cupped under your breast in the shape of a C. If you have small breasts, this may not be necessary after a time, but try the C-hold initially to make sure baby latches on correctly.

Encouraging baby to get a successful latch is the most important part of the process. Stroke her bottom lip with your nipple until she opens her mouth wide and yawn-like. This is called the *rooting reflex*. Insert your nipple into her mouth, and she should instinctively close (latch) onto it.

A proper latch:

✓ Encompasses the entire nipple and most, if not all, of the areola.
✓ Positions baby's nose almost directly on your breast. (She can breathe, don't worry.)

✓ Can be verified by her visible and possibly audible swallowing.

✓ Will not hurt (unless the nipple is in poor condition to begin with).

As your baby nurses, you'll feel a warm tingling that signals the milk ejection reflex (MER) or letdown. The sensation is actually that of milk being released into the sinuses of the breast for easy access by baby. Some women don't always feel the MER, but you'll know that it occurs when your baby suddenly picks up his pace of sucking and swallowing.

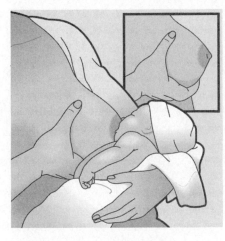

Use the C-hold to support your breast for baby and encourage a proper latch.

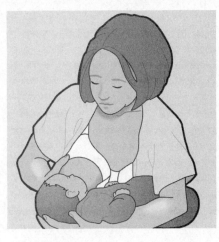

Cross-cradle hold

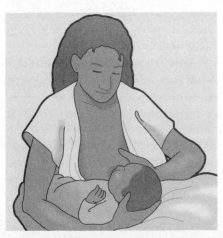

Football clutch hold

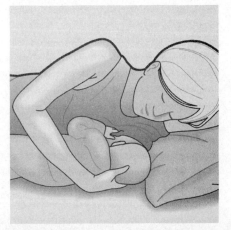

Side lying hold

Supply and Demand System

When the process operates as designed, the more baby nurses, the more milk your breasts produce. A breast that baby has completely drained will produce milk at a faster rate than one that has only been partially emptied. Your milk production takes its cue from baby. So, if your child is premature or ill and isn't nursing, or is latching or sucking ineffectively, your milk supply will adjust downward. A breast pump can help keep the milk flowing until baby is ready to nurse full-time again.

E-QUESTION

I feel like I'm nursing constantly! Is he not getting enough food?
Newborns don't believe much in schedules. In some cases constant nursing in a fussy baby can indicate an insufficient milk supply. But as long as he's growing fine and is having six to eight wet diapers and about three dirty diapers daily, you can be assured he's getting plenty to eat.

Nursing ten to twelve times a day is normal for a newborn. That may seem like a lot, but just bear with it; as the weeks pass and he develops, he'll spend more time exploring and less time eating. In the meantime, his frequent snacks are helping to establish and grow your milk supply, which is great.

Practical Matters

Button-up blouses, shirts with zippers, and other easy-access clothing make nursing easier on a day-to-day basis. There are varieties of nursing bras available; make sure you try them on before purchase to ensure a good fit. You might opt for the comfort of a simple jogging or sports bra that slides up easily, especially if you like the added support of wearing a bra to bed.

Nursing pads for catching leaks before they soak through your shirt are also a must. These come in several different materials and configurations, including cloth, plastic, and disposable. Disposable has the advantage of high absorbency, while cloth can be washed and reused. Accidents do happen, even with pads, and carrying an extra shirt in your bag or car can save you a mortifying moment or two.

Baby's Body and Breastfeeding

Trying to impose a strict feeding schedule on your newborn will result in much heartache and little success. Unless you have multiples, there's really no good reason to start scheduling baby's meals at specific times. If you do have twins or more, you may want to wake them all when one gets up for a feeding in order to get them on a similar routine—but that still doesn't mean feeding by the clock. Only your baby can determine how much he needs to satisfy his tummy, and feeding on demand is the best way to accomplish this.

The health rewards for your nursing child's body and mind are tremendous. Breastmilk improves immunity, is thought to offer protection against certain chronic diseases (for example, type 1 diabetes), is associated with a reduced risk of SIDS, and is easy on baby's digestive system. Clinical studies have also indicated that breastfeeding can enhance cognitive development in small-for-gestational-age (SGA) babies.

So, how long do you breastfeed? From a clinical standpoint, the American Academy of Pediatrics has recommended exclusive breastfeeding for at least 6 months and promotes breastfeeding for a year or longer, as long as both mother and child are still comfortable with the arrangement. The best answer is probably as long as both of you are still enjoying and benefiting from it.

Bottle Basics

If you do choose to bottle-feed, there are literally hundreds of bottle types and nipple configurations on the market to choose from. Figuring out what works and what doesn't is largely trial and error, but there are some factors you can look for:

✓ **Low air flow.** Designs that minimize air or that can be de-aired prior to feeding can reduce baby's gas.

✓ **Convenience.** If saving time is a priority, features like presterilized disposable bag bottles are a big plus.

✓ **Easy to clean.** Pick a bottle with minimal parts, one that looks relatively easy to clean and sterilize.

✓ **Built for baby.** Make sure to start baby with a newborn-style nipple that has a smaller opening so that she doesn't face a formula tidal wave. If her sucking reflex is weak, however, you might have to upgrade to a larger opening.

Both breastfed and bottle-fed babies require regular burping during a meal. You'll quickly pick up your child's cues that a bubble needs bursting; she may arch her back and fuss at the breast or bottle. In the beginning, burping at least twice during a feeding session can help to ensure her comfort.

An infant's tiny stomach can only hold 2 to 4 teaspoons of fluid at birth. Spitting up is his signal that the tank is full. Swallowing air and engaging in too much activity with a full tummy can also cause spitting up. However, if baby's spit-up becomes excessive and forceful (projectile vomiting), or is accompanied by gagging or difficulty swallowing, call your pediatrician immediately. It could be a sign that your baby has a formula intolerance or a gastrointestinal problem.

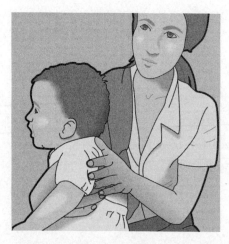

There are several positions you can use to burp baby effectively: seated, over the shoulder, and across the lap.

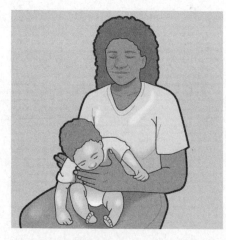

Seated burp position

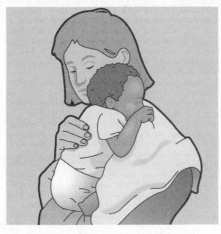 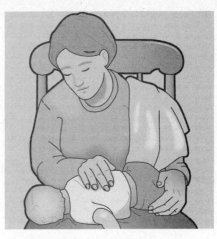

Over the shoulder burp position   Across the lap burp position

Eating Right: For Mom

A pattern of healthy eating in pregnancy will continue to reward you and baby now that you're breastfeeding. Keep up the same routine with healthy food choices and plenty of noncaffeinated fluids (eight to twelve glasses a day). Nursing burns approximately 500 calories per day. Make nutrient-dense choices, including plenty of fruits, vegetables, whole grains, and animal- and plant-based protein foods.

E-ALERT!

If baby becomes fussy after nursing, the cause could be something you ate. Spicy foods can be a trigger, but so can less obvious culprits like milk, grains, and citrus fruits. Skin reactions and congestion can also signal a problem. Keep a food diary to track what foods seem to trigger the reaction, and avoid those that seem to cause problems.

Even though you might be tempted to cut calories drastically in order to get your former figure back, now is not the time to crash diet. Losing weight too quickly can release excessive levels of any toxins, like pesticides and PCBs, that reside in your maternal fat stores and that will consequently pass into breastmilk. Also stay away from extremely low carbohydrate diets right now since they can cause ketosis, a potential danger to a nursing baby.

On Your Mind

Breastfeeding doesn't come naturally to everyone. Ingrained feelings of self-consciousness about your body, of modesty, and of discomfort with the process can inhibit your natural inclination to nurse. When efforts don't go according to plan and the nursing relationship isn't thriving, feelings of inadequacy are common. Seeking assistance, either through coaching or supplemental nutrition, is not a sign of failure but rather of dedication to your child. Breastfeeding in any amount is something to take tremendous pride in.

Breasts: From Form to Function

Where is the right setting to nurse? Wherever your baby is hungry. As long as breastfeeding is done as discreetly as circumstances warrant, any place that's appropriate to take a baby is the right spot.

The prospect of nursing in public might be worrying you. When the time comes, don't think about your exposure; think only of filling your child's stomach. A baby who's really singing for his supper will probably not give you the time to be modest about it, anyway.

Specially designed nursing blankets can improve your cover if you're really self-conscious, although a receiving blanket over the shoulder works as well. If you do use a nursing blanket, make sure it's comfortable and not too hot for baby.

Support from Family and Friends

Breastfeeding doesn't always come naturally and immediately, particularly for first-time moms. Having the support of your friends and family is really important in making it through those first few uncertain and sometimes rocky weeks. Comments like "Why don't you just give her a bottle?" will do nothing but erode your confidence and stress you out. Get your partner's help in deflecting the negativity and justifying your reasons for breastfeeding, and if the bad attitudes continue, just avoid the offender. You don't need it.

A La Leche League International group can also be a steadfast source of support and inspiration and, more important, can offer guidance for your breastfeeding difficulties. Call 1-800-LALECHE for a group in your area, or visit their website at *www.llli.org*.

Lactation Problems

Learning to read baby's body language and hear vocal cues is an acquired art, one that takes time to acclimate to. It's easy to miss hunger signals or mistake them for other needs. For now, familiarize yourself with the warning signs of insufficient feeding. If your baby is having fewer than six wet and three dirty diapers a day, is excessively fussy at the breast, has a sunken fontanel (soft spot), acts lethargic, and is not at or above birth weight by 2 weeks postpartum (or steadily gaining thereafter), he is probably not getting enough milk and needs to see his pediatrician immediately. Fortunately, with some work and a little guidance, you should both be able to get back on track.

Why Your Body Isn't Cooperating

There are dozens of reasons why milk supply or nursing itself may not be making the cut, but most of them can be overcome with patience, special equipment, and/or professional training and guidance.

- **Medications:** Antihistamines, decongestants, contraceptives, and some other medications can have a detrimental effect on milk supply. Talk to your doctor before taking any medication while nursing.
- **Inverted nipples:** If you have inverted nipples, a good latch may be elusive. Breast shields designed to pull out the nipple can help.
- **Prior breast surgery:** Many women nurse successfully after breast surgery, but certain types of breast augmentation (enlargement) or breast reduction surgery do have the potential to hinder your milk supply, depending on how they are performed. Talk to your doctor if you've had breast surgery and are having lactation problems.
- **Hypotrophic breast disease:** Some women have structural problems with the breast tissue that decreases the number of milk-producing

ducts. You may still be able to nurse, but baby might require supplemental feedings. Again, speak with your provider about your options.

- **Retained placental fragment:** Lactation problems can be a sign that a piece of your placenta was retained in delivery. Because this can also cause severe hemorrhage and infection, a suspected retained placenta should be assessed by your provider immediately.
- **Stress:** New motherhood and all its related stressors can inhibit milk supply, and tension can make letdown (milk ejection) difficult. If you're uptight about nursing problems, the cycle perpetuates itself. Try to look forward to nursing as a relaxing, *de*-stressing time.
- **Poor technique:** Letting baby empty one breast before moving on to the next will stimulate milk supply and allow her to reach the fatty and filling hindmilk at the end of her drink.
- **Poor nutrition and hydration:** Good eating habits and plenty of water are essential to your milk-production efforts.
- **Nipple confusion:** The mechanics of drinking from a bottle are very different from those of feeding from the breast. If a bottle is introduced before breastfeeding is well established, it's possible for your baby to develop a preference for it.

Babies born prematurely, those with a poor sucking reflex, or those with a cleft lip or other health problem can have problems nursing initially. If your baby needs supplemental feeding in the hospital for any reason, you can request that it be administered with an eyedropper, syringe, feeding cup, or supplemental feeding system to avoid nipple confusion. You should also talk with your pediatrician and a lactation consultant about adaptive techniques and other options.

Lactation Consultants

A lactation consultant is a health care provider who specializes in breastfeeding support and training. If you're having difficulties with nursing, a consultant can be a huge help in overcoming breastfeeding difficulties. Your ob-gyn or your child's pediatrician can provide a referral if needed. Some large pediatric practices retain lactation consultants on staff.

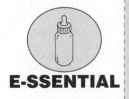

A board-certified lactation consultant will have the designation "IBCLC" (International Board Certified Lactation Consultant) or "IBCLC, RLC" (Registered Lactation Consultant). These means she meets specific eligibility and experience requirements and has passed a board examination administered by the International Board of Lactation Consultant Examiners (IBLCE). Sometimes consultants are nurses who have earned board certification.

Many certified lactation consultants are also La Leche League leaders. Don't overlook the value of La Leche League support if you have no lactation consultant in your area. The organization can be a tremendous source of emotional support as well as practical advice and expertise.

Pump Primer

A breast pump can be useful in ramping up your milk production if you're having supply issues. It's also a great tool for moms heading back to work who want to keep nursing, as well as for mothers of babies who are temporarily unable to nurse for various health reasons.

A pump may be manual (hand powered), battery powered, or a plug-in unit. The hand-powered pumps have the advantage of being inexpensive and portable but can take some getting used to and take longer to empty a breast. They use a piston-like action or a squeeze bulb to create the suction that removes the milk from your breast.

Hospital-grade electric units are probably the most efficient and allow you to pump both breasts at the same time, though they are bulky to transport and costly to purchase. Weekly or monthly rental units are frequently available through lactation consultants, hospital programs, or private businesses. For safety reasons, you will have to purchase a personal kit for use with the rental unit to obtain all the elements that come in contact with your breastmilk, including tubing and bottles. The kit can be used for as long as you plan to pump and usually runs between $20 and $45 monthly for the basics.

Supplemental Feeding

If you're having breastfeeding problems, a supplemental nursing system (SNS) can help you provide baby with added nutrients of pumped breastmilk or formula while still giving the benefits of suckling. A bottle or bag milk reservoir hangs around your neck, and two narrow silicone tubes channel milk flow from the reservoir to your nipple, where the open end of the tube is taped. As baby feeds on both the supplemental milk and breastmilk you're providing, her suckling action further stimulates your milk production.

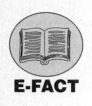

E-FACT

Beyond the immediate physical benefits of helping to speed your postpartum body back into shape, breastfeeding can have long-term benefits for maternal health. Studies have suggested that women who breastfeed have a lower risk of developing premenopausal breast cancer and ovarian cancer and postmenopausal osteoporosis and hip fractures.

Women who are having problems producing enough milk for whatever reason may be able to supplement from a local breastmilk bank if one is nearby. Milk donors are screened for health problems in a process similar to blood-donation screening. Again, a lactation consultant or pediatrician should have further information on what's available in your area.

Mastitis

Mastitis is an infection of the breast that can be caused by a plugged milk duct. If you develop mastitis, you can and should keep nursing. Your baby cannot get ill, and the breastfeeding process will actually help the mastitis resolve itself faster by easing the pain and draining the milk ducts.

Signs of mastitis include:

- Breast is warm to the touch
- Red, tender streaks on the breast
- Pain and swelling
- Fever present

If you develop mastitis, stay on your nursing schedule and try to get sufficient rest to help your body heal. A warm water bottle, warm wet compress, or soak in a hot shower can help to ease the discomfort. If the mastitis doesn't start to clear up in a day or so or begins to worsen, you might need an antibiotic. Your health care provider can advise you as to what medications will be safe for breastfeeding.

Just for Dads

Although it may look easy, breastfeeding can be hard work, particularly the first time out. Your support is vital to this venture. Let your partner know you value this unique gift she's bestowing on your child. Be a voice of support when things get tough, and do what you can to create a warm and welcome environment for your nursing twosome. If the whole process has you bewildered, don't be embarrassed about asking questions.

Getting Comfortable with Breastfeeding

Be honest. Somewhere in the back of your mind (or perhaps unabashedly front and center), you were a little freaked out at the notion of your partner as food source. If you weren't, more power to you, but it's normal to need a little time to adjust. Learning more about how beneficial breastfeeding is for your new baby can help increase your comfort level.

When you're both up to sex again, try to respect your partner's feelings about touching on the feeding zone. Nipple soreness, leaking milk, and breast sensitivity might have her feeling better left alone. Or she could be willing while you are hesitant, given whose mouth was there last. Whatever the situation, it's important that you each get your current viewpoint out in the open so that no one's feelings are hurt. Your outlook may evolve over time, or you may both decide to focus on other sources of pleasure.

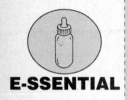

One thing you'll quickly learn about infant timing is that you'll be interrupted in the heat of passion at least once. And when your partner returns from nursing baby, realize that switching gears from nurturing mommy to adventurous sex kitten can be a tall order to fill. Don't force an uncomfortable and awkward situation if the moment has passed for either of you.

Remember that you won't have an infant forever; making adjustments to your sex life is just one of the many detours that parenting brings.

Getting In On the Act

You're probably grateful for your gender at those middle-of-the-night feedings, but during the day it might be nice to be able to feed baby once in a while. Just because your partner is nursing doesn't cut you out of the feeding picture completely. At some point you will want to familiarize baby with a bottle of breastmilk, in case mom's absence requires feeding her expressed (pumped) milk. To avoid any nipple confusion, breastfeeding should be well established first.

Once a bottle is introduced, you can do the honors for a regular feeding if your partner has other obligations or perhaps in order to allow her to get some much-needed sleep at night. Some babies are hesitant to take a bottle from mom when they know her nice warm breast is just an arm's reach away, so your fatherly presence is necessary for this task.

Bringing Baby Home

The first days at home with your new family are fun but challenging. Your body is going through some intense physical changes, and you're adjusting to a brand new way of living—affecting everything from your sleeping patterns to when and how you leave the house. And if you thought those hormonal changes that pregnancy brought are now finished—well, think again. Enjoy this special time of getting acquainted and settling into your new lifestyle.

Your Body Postpartum

From the moment your child slides out of your body, a transformation as dramatic as pregnancy begins. Right at delivery you drop around 10 to 15 pounds of baby, placenta, amniotic fluid, and lochia. Lochia is vaginal discharge of blood, mucus, and tissue.

By the tenth day postpartum, your incredible shrinking uterus contracts to one-twentieth of its prelabor size, and the cervix is closed once again. Afterpains, similar to menstrual cramps, and a steady discharge of lochia indicate that the uterus is returning to normal. The lochia flow continues up to 6 weeks, but the afterpains will probably stop several days after delivery (although nursing may continue to stimulate them periodically). Never use tampons to control lochia flow because of the risk of infection.

Your perineal area may continue to be sore for a few weeks, particularly when you need to relieve yourself. Take your peri bottle from the hospital home with you, and keep it in the bathroom for regular use. A hot water bottle and occasional cold packs can also ease pain and swelling. If sitting is uncomfortable, you can purchase a foam donut at a medical supply store and use it in your chair. Most stitches dissolve within a week, and external ones may fall out. Pelvic-floor exercises (Kegels) can help speed up the healing process.

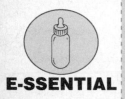

E-SSENTIAL

Lochia flow is heavy and bright red at first, but the color gradually changes to pink and then yellow or brown; the flow is reduced significantly within 10 to 14 days. If bright red lochia occurs after that time, it can mean that you are doing too much too soon.

As your body drops tissues and fluids and decreases its cardiovascular volume, your metabolism can seem completely out of whack. Vaginally, you might feel a little looser in general. Your vaginal skin is quite elastic and is stretched out from the birth. Exercise and time will help it return to a firmer state.

Constipation is another common postpartum problem, primarily because of the loss of abdominal muscle tone and painkillers that can slow your digestive processes. Plenty of water, movement, and high-fiber foods should help. If you have had a C-section, your incision might also make you hesitant to bear down very hard. Supporting it with a rolled-up towel can help. A stool softener may be prescribed as well. If you are breastfeeding, check with your practitioner before taking any medication.

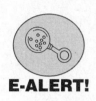

E-ALERT!

Although sex may be the last thing on your mind right now, if you aren't up to a return to the delivery room in 9 or 10 short months, get back on a contraceptive routine now before the mood strikes. Your doctor can give you a prescription before you leave the hospital, if necessary.

Your breasts will be tender as you deal with engorgement. Women who aren't planning on nursing find that fully drying up their milk supply can be a somewhat uncomfortable process. Wear a tight bra, try ice packs to ease discomfort, and avoid any unnecessary stimulation. If you do breastfeed, sore nipples and other discomforts can plague you as you adjust to this new routine.

Recovering after a Cesarean

When you've had a C-section, you're recovering from major surgery and need to treat yourself accordingly. Sleep when baby sleeps, and stay away from strenuous activity and heavy lifting (nothing heavier than baby, as a general rule). Use a bed pillow or a nursing pillow (Boppy) to hold your baby without pressuring your incision. Pain medication may be prescribed; if you're breastfeeding, talk to your doctor about judicious use.

Your doctor will recommend 6 weeks of rest and recuperation (within limits—you are a new mom, after all), and you'll be advised not to drive during that time as well. Second or subsequent C-section moms might recover a bit quicker, just because they know what to expect and treat themselves accordingly. Above all, don't push yourself or you'll set your recovery back even further.

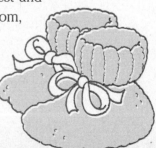

Baby's Body: An Operator's Manual

Your baby will actually lose weight as she starts out in life, but she should be back up to birth weight by her 2-week checkup. Thereafter she may put on a pound every 2 weeks, doubling her birth weight by her 4th month. Premature babies sometimes grow a little slower, but most eventually catch up.

Your baby's eyesight is a bit hazy, although she can see you fairly clearly when you hold her 7 to 10 inches away from your face. Studies show that she knows your voice well from listening to it in the womb, and she prefers to hear it to a stranger's voice.

Your newborn arrives with a variety of natural reflexes or involuntary ways of moving:

- **Palmar (grasping) reflex.** When you touch your baby's open hand, she'll make a fist around your finger.
- **Rooting reflex.** If you stroke her cheek, her head will turn toward your touch. This reflex helps the bleary-eyed newborn find her food source, and you can use it to guide her to the breast or bottle.
- **Sucking reflex.** Once at the breast or bottle, baby's sucking reflex takes over as she automatically sucks on anything put in her mouth.
- **Startle (Moro) reflex.** When baby is startled, he will thrust his arms and legs out, arch his back, then quickly pull arms and legs in again.
- **Babinski reflex.** Stroking baby's foot makes him spread his toes and flex his foot.
- **Stepping reflex.** Hold your baby up with your hands under his armpits so that his feet are touching a firm surface. He will lift his feet up and down like he is about to take baby steps.
- **Tonic neck reflex.** When placed on his back, baby turns his head to the right and makes fists with his hands.
- **Blinking.** The reflex of closing his eyes when they are exposed to bright light, air, or another stimulus is one involuntary reaction that baby will keep for the rest of his life.

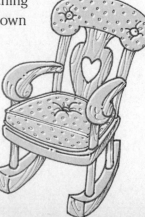

From Soft Spot to Curled Toes

The bones of baby's skull are not yet fused together, and unless you have had a cesarean delivery, your baby's head may look a bit, well, pointy. This cone-headed appearance is the result of pressure in the birth canal and will round out within a few days after birth. There are four small areas on your baby's head where the skull bones have not yet joined; these are called *fontanels* (*soft spots*). Three of these fontanels fuse within the first 4 months of life, but the longest lasting and most visible of these—the diamond-shaped area on the top of the head called the *anterior fontanel*—can take up to 18 months to close. Many a curious sibling has reached out to jab this pulsating spot, much to his parent's horror. Don't get too concerned; your baby's brain is well protected by a tough membrane called the *dura mater*.

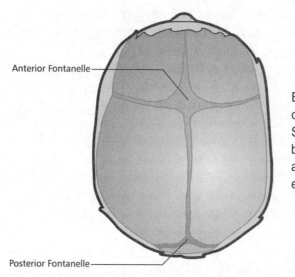

Baby's soft spot is called a fontanelle. She has a total of four, but only the anterior and posterior are easily located.

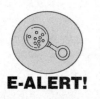

E-ALERT!

A normal fontanel is slightly curved in and soft yet firm to the touch. A deeply sunken soft spot can indicate dehydration, and a fontanel that bulges could be a sign of increased pressure in the brain from fluid buildup or hemorrhage. Both warrant an immediate call to your pediatrician. Keep in mind that crying can make the fontanel appear swollen.

The eye color your baby has at birth may change later in infancy or childhood. This is due to the ongoing production of the hormone melanin.

Baby's Skin

Your newborn's soft-as-butter skin may have some imperfections at first. Post-term babies are more likely to have some peeling, while preterm babies can still be sporting a substantial amount of lanugo and vernix. Although the vernix is fairly well rubbed off by the time you bring baby home, you may continue to find it in his creases and crevices until his first real bath. The lanugo will rub off over the next few weeks.

Baby may also be wearing one or more birthmarks on his birthday suit, including:

- **Salmon patches or "stork bites."** Red marks on the eyelids, forehead, and at the very back of the nape of the neck usually fade and disappear over time.
- **Hemangiomas (strawberry birthmarks).** These red, slightly raised marks can increase in size but may shrink and be gone by age 5.
- **Café au lait spots.** Light-brown birthmarks. Very rarely, large numbers of these birthmarks can be a sign of medical conditions. Talk to your child's doctor if you have any concerns.
- **Mongolian spots.** Dark-blue to blue-green spots on the buttocks or lower back are most common in African American, Native American, and Asian newborns, and many fade over time.
- **Port wine stains.** These bright-red or purple marks are considered to be more permanent. Laser removal is an option in later life if they are located in a prominent spot.
- **Milia.** Little whiteheads called *milia* are common on newborns, especially around the nose, and may come and go during the first few days.
- **Petechiae.** These are red-to-purple pinpoints that you may see on your baby's face from the trauma of coming down the birth canal. These will disappear in a few days.

The Umbilical Cord

Baby's umbilical cord stump looks just like it sounds—a dark, dried-up protrusion. Since it is basically dead tissue, it is black in color. You'll be instructed to clean it regularly and keep it dry to prevent breakage and bleeding. Keep an eye out for signs of infection, such as pus or inflammation. Within 2 weeks or so the stump will fall off, and your baby's perfect little bellybutton will be revealed.

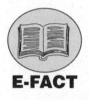

E-FACT

Your baby, boy or girl, may have swollen breasts that actually leak milk. This milk, known in folk medicine as "witch's milk," is the product of your pregnancy hormones at work on your newborn. Avoid massaging the area because this can trigger an abscess. The breasts will return to normal size within a few days.

Genitals

Before your partner congratulates himself too heartily on his well-endowed son, you might want to break the news that this is probably just a passing phenomenon. Newborn boys and girls are often born with swollen genitals, again due to the effects of your pregnancy hormones working on them. Girls can even have a bit of mucus discharge, possibly blood-tinged, from their vaginas.

Fingernails and Toenails

Baby's tiny curled fingers and toes usually emerge in need of a manicure. Growing for several months in the womb, they are typically long and ragged. The thought of trimming such tiny appendages might fill you with dread, but it's not as hard as you think. Just make sure you have the right tools (infant-sized clippers) and try to trim while baby is sleeping (if you'd like to avoid wrestling with a moving target). If you still can't seem to cut the nails, bring your clippers with you to your 2-week pediatrician appointment and ask for pointers.

Sleeping Like a Baby

In the beginning it will seem like your little one is sleeping quite a bit. In fact, she's snoozing up to 18 hours a day. If she's your first, you might be crouched outside her door waiting to run in and get some quality playtime at the first rustle. (Second-time parents, on the other hand, count down the minutes to naptime.) Although her sleep patterns, which involve 4-hour stretches of snoozing, won't have a huge effect on your day schedule, they're going to hit you hard at night. She'll be waking up to be fed several times an evening for at least the first 3 months.

Remember to always place your baby on his back when laying him down for a nap or bedtime. Back sleeping has been shown to reduce the incidence of sudden infant death syndrome (SIDS). Make sure baby's crib is clear of stuffed animals, quilts, pillows, and other soft bedding when he heads to bed.

Postpartum Depression

Feeling down is a common postpartum emotion that typically passes in a few weeks. For many women, however, these feelings go beyond the basic baby blues and signal a more serious depressive or endocrine disorder.

The Baby Blues

The majority of new mothers experience what is commonly known as *the baby blues*, a short-lived period of mild depression that appears in up to 85 percent of postpartum women. A severe shortage of sleep, disappointment with the birth experience, seesawing hormone levels, anxieties about baby's health and well-being, and shaky confidence in your own parenting skills all can lead to feelings of sadness or inadequacy. Fortunately, most cases of the blues resolve themselves between a few days to 2 weeks after birth, as balance returns to the new mother's life.

When It's More than the Blues

More serious is postpartum depression (PPD), which occurs in about 10 to 15 percent of new mothers and can drag on for up to a year. If you're experiencing one or more of the following symptoms, talk to your doctor about PPD:

- Feelings of extreme sadness and inexplicable crying jags
- Lack of pleasure in things you would normally enjoy
- Trouble concentrating
- Excessive worrying about the baby or, conversely, a lack of interest in the baby
- Feelings of low self-esteem
- Decreased appetite

Fortunately, PPD can be effectively treated with counseling and/or antidepressant drugs, so ask your doctor for a referral to a mental health professional. Even if you're breastfeeding, you have medication options; there are several antidepressant drugs on the market that are thought to have minimal effect on nursing infants. A number of studies involving sertraline (Zoloft), for example, found that even though the drug passes into breastmilk, the levels it reaches in the nursing infant are clinically insignificant, in some cases too low even to be detected in standard laboratory blood tests.

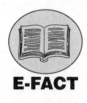

E-FACT

Several studies have indicated that low postpartum hemoglobin levels (iron-deficiency anemia) increase the risk of postpartum depression. Ask your doctor about your blood hemoglobin levels, especially if you have a history of iron-deficiency anemia. Increasing dietary iron intake and taking daily iron supplements will improve hemoglobin levels and may alleviate depressive symptoms.

Safety cannot be guaranteed, however; studies on how antidepressants affect a breastfed child in the long term are not available. On the other hand, clinical research has demonstrated a measurable detrimental effect on children of depressed mothers when PPD goes untreated. Each woman must evaluate the risks of treatment versus the benefits when deciding whether drug therapy is right for her.

Postpartum Psychosis

An estimated one in every 1,000 women experiences a severe form of PPD known as *postpartum psychosis* (*puerperal psychosis*). Symptoms include hallucinations, delusions, fantasies of hurting oneself or others, insomnia, and turbulent mood swings. Postpartum psychosis is a medical emergency that needs immediate treatment and usually hospitalization. The good news is that with proper medical care, full recovery is expected.

Thyroid Problems

Thyroid problems are fairly common after childbirth, but the symptoms can be confused with other postpartum conditions. Milk supply difficulties, extreme fatigue, hair loss, depression, mood changes, problems losing weight or unusually rapid weight loss, heart palpitations, menstrual irregularities, and sleep disorders are all common signs of postpartum thyroid conditions.

Some women have temporary postpartum hyperthyroidism (an overactive thyroid), with the result of weight loss, diarrhea, racing heart, anxiety, and other symptoms of a revved-up metabolism. Your doctor may prescribe drugs to ease symptoms, although this condition often resolves itself quickly.

Other women can develop temporary postpartum hypothyroidism (an underactive thyroid), resulting in fatigue, weight gain, constipation, depression, and other symptoms of a slowed-down metabolism. Again, medication may be prescribed depending on the severity of symptoms, and frequently the thyroid returns to normal within 6 months to a year after the birth.

New mothers with a family or personal history of autoimmune or thyroid disease can benefit from routine thyroid testing in the first month postpartum. It can be hard to tell what's normal after having a baby, but if any of the aforementioned symptoms become debilitating, a thyroid test can quickly rule out or diagnose a thyroid problem.

Women who experience temporary postpartum thyroid problems are at a higher risk of developing thyroid disease later in life and should talk to their doctor about regular follow-up screening.

Adjusting to Your New Schedule

Many aspects of your life are different now that you are a parent. You probably feel that your priorities are altered since you have a little one to think about. But taking time to care for yourself is equally important.

Bonding with Baby

These early weeks and months are a precious time of mother and child getting to know each other and of your building confidence in mothering. Yet after your baby has cried for 20 minutes straight and you still haven't guessed what's wrong (is she hungry, dirty, tired, colicky, gassy?), you might start to wonder about your mothering abilities. Trust yourself. Although it takes time to learn baby's language, the patience and persistence you invest in decoding her signals will pay off. You'll crack the code eventually, and in the process you'll establish a bond of trust and communication that lasts a lifetime.

Sleep, or Lack of It

People told you how tired you would be when baby arrived, but after 3 months of uncomfortable, interrupted sleep leading up to the delivery, you thought you were well prepared. Surprise. You feel like the walking dead and crave sleep constantly. Your baby will sleep through the night eventually. In the meantime, give yourself a break by splitting night duties with your spouse or significant other. Even if you're breastfeeding, if baby is in another room your partner can help out by retrieving him. Also remember the new mom credo: Nap when the baby naps. Forget laundry; forget dishes. You need your rest more than a clean house right now.

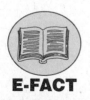

E-FACT

The term *bonding* was coined in 1976 by Drs. Marshall Klaus and John Kennell, two professors of pediatrics who published the pioneering work *Maternal-Infant Bonding*. Klaus and Kennell introduced the theory that close, personal contact between mother and baby was essential in the first 30 to 60 minutes after birth to build the foundation for a healthy attachment.

And if you've only slept 3 hours the previous night, between bouts of calming a fussy baby? Don't get behind the wheel of a car before you get some adequate shuteye. Extreme fatigue slows your reaction time, and you run a very real risk of falling asleep behind the wheel. The National Highway Traffic Safety Administration (NHTSA) estimates that driving while drowsy is responsible for at least 100,000 automobile accidents annually between the hours of 10 P.M. and 6 A.M.

Setting Priorities

You aren't going to be able to do it all. If you try to keep up your preparenthood schedule in addition to your new motherhood duties, something or someone has to give. Usually it's your sanity. Let matters that just aren't that important, usually anything in the domesticity arena, lag a bit. As the motivational gurus like to say: work smarter, not harder. Buy the birthday cake at the bakery instead of baking it yourself. Use a delivery service to get your groceries. Pay the kid down the block to mow the lawn.

Don't Forget to Have Fun

Once you get past the fatigue, the uncertainties, and the occasional frustrations, being a new mom can be incredibly entertaining. You have a legitimate excuse to play, explore, rhyme, sing, and generally revisit your childhood. You have an adoring little person who hangs on your every word and movement and loves you unconditionally. And you get to witness all of his incredible firsts as your tiny miracle learns to smile, roll over, crawl, and eventually walk and talk. A year from now, this postpartum time will be a distant memory. Treasure it while it's here.

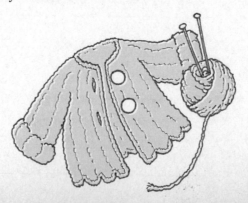

The Rest of the Family

Obviously, you aren't doing this alone. Even if you're a single mom, you have people in your life who care for you and baby. Involve your family or those around you, and baby and you will benefit.

Support

You might learn that your mother really does know a thing or two. It's amazing to watch her and your dad soothe and burp their grandchild like they've been doing it forever. Just like riding a bike, apparently. And they often have a baby-wrangling trick or two up their sleeves that will make your life easier. Every family relationship is different, of course, but witnessing the ones who raised you cuddle and care for the child that you now nurture instills a sense of connectivity and completeness, as if your life has come full circle. Now just hope that all those prophecies they made about "hoping you have a child just like you" don't come to fruition!

Neighbors and friends will likely call, both to check on the new addition and to find out whether they can do anything for you. One simple rule: Take all help that is offered. Don't feel guilty, and don't feel like you're putting anyone out. They wouldn't offer if they didn't mean it. And even if they did offer just because they thought they should, they'll think twice next time—won't they?

E-QUESTION

What's the best way to introduce our dog to the new baby?
Because animals learn from scents, some new parents bring home a receiving blanket from the hospital and give it to their dog to get acquainted. Let the first meeting between dog and baby be a gradual and calm affair with only immediate family present. And always supervise every encounter between your baby and pet.

Sibling Rivalry

Give your older child a chance to bond with baby on the sibling level. Older kids frequently get a kick out of holding, feeding, and protecting their new little sibling. Children who are preschool age or younger might have a more difficult time accepting this drain on their parents' attention. Some tips to promote sibling harmony:

- If you're breastfeeding, establish a family routine of a snack or story when baby nurses to make it a special time for all.
- Involve your child in age-appropriate baby care. Helping with a bath or diaper change can be just the incentive he needs to relish his new big-brother role.
- Try to arrange some special parental one-on-one time. Even if you just have a quick story during baby's nap, try to have a designated time in which your firstborn is the star of the show.
- Tell your older child stories about her babyhood. Hearing how she threw strained peas at daddy or wore her very ripe diaper as a hat will have her in stitches and can help her relate a bit better to this odd little creature.
- Don't use the baby as an excuse. If children constantly hear "we can't do that because the baby is sleeping," guess whom they start to blame for the new crimp in their social lives? Instead, provide baby-friendly alternatives when you have to say no: "We can't go swimming today, but we can go for a walk to the park." And arrange some time to take your "big kid" someplace he's been dying to go without a baby sibling in tow.

Daddy Time

Don't hog the baby. Make sure that daddy gets his own chance at bonding time. With a constant flow of visitors and your many hours clocked on baby duty, he may be feeling left out. Both he and your child need time alone together. Getting out and moving on a short walk is good exercise for you right now and a healthy way to clear your head after a day of talking in baby talk. Hand the reins over, without direction or judgment if at all possible, and give dad a chance to run the show.

Just for Dads

Finally, a chance for hands-on parenting. Perhaps you still find yourself feeling outside the family circle. Are you hesitant to jump into this foreign world or feeling like there isn't much left for you to handle? Remember that it is just as important for you to forge a strong bond with your child as it is for your significant other. Start small if it helps your confidence level. Even a task as simple as bundling your baby is an opportunity for relationship building.

Developing Your Own Daddy Style

There is more than one right way to change a diaper, warm a bottle, and calm a fussy baby. You will have your own way of doing things, and that is more than all right: that's good for your whole family. It teaches your baby that there are differences between mommy and daddy, and she will learn what to expect from your unique parenting style.

Don't be a bystander. If you feel like you're getting the brushoff when it comes to baby, let your partner know. She may be so preoccupied with new motherhood and other concerns that she isn't even aware of her behavior. Offer to take charge of regular tasks like bathing. If you feel a little shaky, ask her to stay within shouting distance so that you can get help if need be. But remember, the only reason she seems to handle baby so effortlessly is practice. That's all you need as well.

Set up a date for just baby and you—a trip to the park, a neighborhood walk, even some playtime in the backyard will do. Your partner can have some badly needed time to herself, and you can stretch your caregiving wings.

Male Bonding

You are smitten, preoccupied, utterly in love with this new person in your life, and he with you. The feeling is aptly called *engrossment*, and it's your version of dad-to-baby bonding. Despite societal expectations and dated clichés of fatherhood, men can be just as nurturing and loving as parents and caregivers as women. So, dote on your child, spend time with him, play with him, diaper him, tickle him, and do anything else that comes naturally.

Easing Back into Intimacy

Once baby arrived and your partner got at least a semblance of her former self back, you thought sex would quickly follow. It hasn't. When you consider reality, it shouldn't surprise you: Quick snatches of sleep, a sore and still-recovering body, and all the concerns and anxieties that come with new motherhood are putting the damper on intimacy yet again.

If she is the primary caregiver at home with baby right now, there are probably days when she doesn't even manage to get dressed until well past noon. Having dried spit-up in your hair and baby poop on your pajama bottoms doesn't make you feel much like getting romantic. She needs a little empathy, TLC, and pampering (yes, again) to get back into a more amorous state of mind. Work on supporting her, helping with household duties, and encouraging her rest and recovery. Once her basic needs and responsibilities are met, she can spend a little more time on the two of you.

Back in the Swing of Things

Although it seems overwhelming at first, it won't take you long to get the parenting basics down and settle into your new and demanding role. Making career and family choices, building new and stronger relationships with your partner, and getting back in tune with your body are all priorities during the first year postpartum. That and watching your newborn learn, discover the world, and develop into her own little person.

Getting Your Body Back

Another time-tested motherhood maxim is worth repeating: It took 9 months for you to become this size, so give yourself at least that much time to get your body back. Actually, giving yourself a year is more realistic if you factor in a 3-month transitional period after the birth of your child. As you hammer out a routine wherein you and baby manage to get dressed and bathed before dinnertime, little time is left for structured exercise in these early days.

Set realistic goals for weight loss. Losing weight too rapidly can actually be dangerous for you as well as for your child if you're breastfeeding, and in fact you need to continue to consume some extra calories if you're nursing.

Many women find it difficult to lose weight in the postpartum period because they're working hard, nursing, and are sleep deprived. The time crunch all new mothers face can make a sensible, nutritious diet and a regular exercise regimen seem like a monumental task. Start slow and easy, and a pattern will form.

Exercise

Once you have your doctor's okay to get moving again, start slowly. Even if you were a fitness fanatic throughout pregnancy, you'll still have to ramp back up to reach your former conditioning level. Attend to your body. If you start experiencing bright-red lochia discharge, it's a signal that you're probably doing too much, too fast.

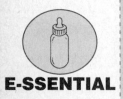

E-SSENTIAL

Stretch marks—your merit badges of pregnancy—are not going to disappear with exercise. If they haven't already, they will probably fade to barely noticeable silvery squiggles, and probably no one but you will even recognize them. But if you are self-conscious, studies have shown that both Retin-A and laser treatment are effective methods for banishing them.

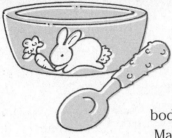

If you've have had a C-section, it's really important to stick to doctor's orders regarding exercise. Most providers recommend at least a 6-week recovery time, but talk to your doctor about guidelines specific to you. Don't risk your health by starting a full-fledged campaign to recover your prepregnancy body before that allotted time.

Many new moms find that their biggest challenge to regular exercise is just finding time. Try these tips for squeezing it in:

✓ **Keep it simple.** Programs with steps, balls, bands, saucers, and other gear are probably not for you right now if you're just getting started. You haul around enough stuff just keeping baby clean and well fed. Don't add to it.

✓ **Baby steps.** Start small. Commit to 20 or 30 minutes a day of movement, and work your way up from there.

✓ **Pencil yourself in.** Set a regular schedule for your partner or a babysitter to care for baby, then use the time to get out and get moving.

✓ **Be flexible.** Do away with the all-or-nothing attitude. If you can't get to the gym one day, take a brisk walk or bike ride instead. Every little bit helps.

✓ **Buddy system.** If you're lucky enough to have a friend or neighbor nearby who is also a new mom, pair up. You can cheer each other on and commiserate.

✓ **Get baby in the act.** Get a jogging stroller and start a regular walking schedule, or simply incorporate more activity into your play. The park is a great place to start.

✓ **Join a gym.** Many health clubs and community programs (like the YMCA) have nursery areas for their members. This might be an option for you if financially feasible. Do take the opportunity to watch the staff in action before enrolling.

Eating Right

Exercise and good nutrition together are the best way to lose your pregnancy weight. If you established healthy eating patterns in pregnancy, you're ahead of the game. If not, now is as good a time as any to get started.

Breastfeeding shouldn't change your diet substantially. You need an increase of around 500 calories daily to meet milk-production needs while you establish your milk supply, but you can reduce that to 100–200 calories daily once you and baby settle into your new routine. You may also want to continue your daily prenatal vitamin. Talk to your doctor for specific guidance.

Another big benefit of breastfeeding can be a faster postpartum rate of weight loss. Although every mom is different, nursing helps you drop the fat stores you collected in pregnancy for the very purpose of lactation. Your body works hard to produce milk and also burns calories faster as a result.

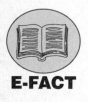

E-FACT

Many childhood education programs and community centers offer parent-and-child exercise classes, so check out this fun way to teach your child healthy fitness habits early on. Or try one of the many child-parent exercise videos on the market.

Typically, as long as you're choosing your foods wisely, you can let your stomach be your guide. Drink plenty of fluids. They're essential to keeping you well hydrated, and nursing has a tendency to make you thirsty. Having a glass of water or other noncaffeinated beverage each time baby nurses is a good ritual to establish proper fluid intake. The restrictions of pregnancy (no alcohol, tobacco, drugs) should also be continued throughout breastfeeding.

Making Up Sleep Deficits

Sleep is also an important factor in getting your old self back. If you're too tired to function, exercise has little appeal. You may find yourself opting for a fast-food fix for dinner instead of taking the time and energy to prepare healthier fare. And your health can suffer as well. Sleep deprivation affects the immune system; chronic sleep loss has been linked to decreases in growth hormone (responsible for bone-marrow growth and tissue healing), increased insulin resistance, and a decline in tumor necrosis factor (natural killer cells, cancer- and virus-fighting agents). Mood disorders such as depression can also be made worse by insufficient sleep. And, of course, you're already aware of the zombielike brain fog that those all-nighters bring. In short, sleep loss is a real health hazard. You can't run on empty forever.

E-ALERT!

If you had gestational diabetes during pregnancy, you have a higher risk of developing type 2 diabetes. The American Diabetes Association recommends that your blood glucose levels be tested 6 to 12 weeks after pregnancy. You should also continue to have lifelong screenings at 3-year intervals.

So, how do you get it back? Take naps whenever possible, of course, and consider a little creative shift work. If your child is not nursing when he wakes in the middle of the night, you can alternate night-shift baby duty with dad so that at least one of you has unbroken slumber every other day. This is even possible with breastfeeding if you've introduced a bottle to baby; just pump breastmilk the evening prior so that your presence won't be necessary. You may get a protest the first time dad attempts to put baby back to sleep with a rubber nipple instead of with mom's warm breast, but don't give up on the first try. Sometimes a little adjustment period is all that's necessary to ease into this new schedule.

The Incredible Changing Baby

Your infant will reach new milestones in such dizzying succession that you'll be convinced you have a prodigy on your hands. Watch her transform from a floppy-necked, bleary-eyed newborn to an active and alert infant in a matter of months. As she starts to become more aware of her surroundings and to interact more with you and her environment, your providing encouragement, stimulation, and patience will help her thrive.

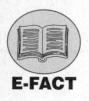

Preemie growth and development are assessed based on the age from estimated delivery date instead of actual birth date for the first 2 years of life. So, a 4-month-old infant who was born 1 month prematurely would be assessed for her attainment of 3-month developmental milestones and size guidelines instead of for 4-month milestones.

Your pediatrician will give you an idea of appropriate developmental milestones as your baby grows. Remember, these are just averages, and some may be reached earlier or later than others. Every child grows at his own pace. The main function of milestones is to serve as a screening tool; if baby is lagging on many, it can be a sign of a problem, but one or two delays is typically no cause for concern.

Your Career

As maternity leave approaches the end, you might find yourself facing decisions you hadn't anticipated. The thought of leaving baby with a caregiver could be tearing you apart. Conversely, if you've put your career on hold for now to stay home with your child, you may find yourself missing the mental challenges and feelings of self-validation that work provides. Changing your mind, either for or against a career outside the home, is not a terrible thing.

If You Decide Not to Return to Work

You had every intention of going back to the office after maternity leave was over, but you never expected to fall so deeply in love, not just with your child but also with motherhood. Or perhaps the thought of leaving your vulnerable little infant with someone outside his immediate family has you rethinking your options.

Financial concerns are an issue, of course. In many cases the costs of child care and career-related expenses like dry-cleaning bills and transportation costs come close to offsetting the difference between a one- and two-income lifestyle. There may be a middle ground, such as picking up part-time work to cover the spread. Or having dad stay home may be a viable alternative. Sit down and hash out the numbers with your partner. Adaptability and creative thinking can reveal a solution.

Going Back to Work

One of the hardest parts of new parenthood is heading back to the office. Getting up to speed on projects and procedures, handling the deluge from managers and coworkers who were basically lost without you, and fighting to stay off the mommy track—all while worrying about how your child is adapting to her new care arrangements—that's a tall order to handle. If you can arrange it, try easing back into employment with a reduced schedule (for example, half days or 3 days a week) to smooth the transition for you and your child.

Your best source of leads for good child care is other moms in your life who share your values and viewpoints on child rearing. You can narrow down your list to facilities that have adequate staffing (for infants, this is generally a minimum of one provider to every three babies), a stimulating and child-friendly environment, and caring and nurturing staff.

Making Time for Yourself and Using It

When your career comes back in the picture, daily life can accelerate to a frenzied pace. Don't just pay lip service to making time for yourself; do it. Even though it can be incredibly tempting to cancel your grown-up plans in favor of lazing around at home or getting some extra household chores done, don't give in to the temptation. You'll find that time alone or with adult company (work doesn't count) is a great recharger. Some tips for following through:

- **Buy tickets to something.** You're less likely to bow out if there's money involved.
- **Invite a friend.** Again, committing to a date and event will make you more likely to follow through.
- **Pick something with a payoff.** A shopping trip to the one place you know that has

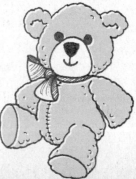

that hard-to-find Christmas gift you've been searching for can get you up and out.

- **Schedule a sitter right off the bat.** A short respite from child care, particularly if it leaves baby in the hands of a doting relative who would be sorely disappointed if you canceled, is a good incentive to keep your date with yourself.

A Whole New Family

Beyond your new parenting relationship, other family dynamics have definitely changed since baby's arrival. You and your partner may find yourselves hard pressed for time to spend together, with practical concerns like money more of an issue as you learn how to adjust your lifestyle and income for three (or more). And if you have some specific plans for a family, you could even be thinking about pregnancy again.

Intimacy Issues

Perhaps for the first time in months, you are rediscovering your interest in sex. Of course, your little one could be putting a damper on things unwittingly; remember that she is bound to interrupt you in the height of passion at least once. Flexibility is key to having a healthy sex life with kids around. Grab time together when it presents itself, and follow these tips for rekindling the fire:

- **No baby talk.** Calling each other mommy and daddy around the kids is fine, but this can really kill the mood if it slips out in other circumstances.
- **Take it slow and easy.** Give both of you time to rediscover each other. There may be a learning curve with your postpregnancy body.
- **Love yourself.** It's hard to enjoy lovemaking if you're self-conscious about the way you look. Accept the state of your body whatever it is, and instead see it as a visible manifestation of the miracle of your baby.

- **Quiet, please.** You don't need to turn the baby monitor up to eleven. Hearing every tiny baby sigh is a turnoff. Just turn the monitor down and open your door instead; if she wakes up, she will let you know.

Financial Planning

By now you've gotten a feel of how much it costs to care for your new family member, and you're either pleasantly surprised or in a panic. If the former, pat yourself on the back and consider saving your extra pennies in a new college fund for your child (a financial advisor can help you explore your options).

If you're in the panic category, take a deep breath and try to pinpoint the problem. Are the extra expenses coming from baby gadgetry and other non-essential purchases or from necessities like diapers and wipes? A budget is really important in assessing the family finances now, so if you didn't create one during pregnancy, now is the time to start. There are places to cut back if you look for them. Finally, if you find yourself hopelessly in debt no matter how you look at the situation, you need to see a reputable credit counselor to get back on a positive financial footing.

The Next Time Around

The first birthday is usually the time when everyone starts asking about a sibling for your "big" kid. When you're done rolling your eyes and laughing, you start to actually give the notion some serious consideration. Are you ready to do it all over again?

Beyond physical readiness, how will you know? Suddenly the sight of another woman in her 9th month brings about warm memories instead of enormous relief that it's not you, and you seem to have forgotten the perils of pregnancy and pain of childbirth.

If you're sold on a family with kids close enough in age to play and go to the same school together, you may be ready to start a bit sooner. Try to give your body time to recover so that you don't cheat yourself and your next child out of a healthy pregnancy. A 2-year breather from birth to birth is ideal.

Just for Dads

Are you waiting for life to get back to normal? Stop right there. This is the new normal: Take nothing for granted, be ready to change plans at a moment's notice, and learn to multitask. In other words, if you're a creature of habit and routine, you need to adjust your way of looking at the world.

The Night Shift

If you work a regular day job and then come home to play with and care for baby, it's easy to start burning the candle at both ends. You stay up later and later after baby's bedtime to get things done or to just unwind and end up getting only a few hours of sleep on the clock before your child is up for another feeding. This is bad for your health and your sanity. Split the night shift with your partner so that you're at least getting all your sleep half the time.

Making Adjustments

Life as a father is full of compromise. The library you and your wife started is now a playroom, and the motorcycle you've been lusting after has been shelved (even with a sidecar, it just wouldn't be the same). You planned on spending your weekend watching the NFL draft, but reality strikes and you end up doing laps around the house with a sick and fussy baby instead. Yet instead of envying your childless friends who are at home awaiting the next pick, you look at your child and wish you could take the hurt away and be sick for her instead. Congratulations: You are a father.

Special Concerns in Pregnancy

The vast majority of American women have an uncomplicated pregnancy. While it's natural to worry about things like miscarriage, preterm birth, and genetic defects, dwelling on every possible thing that could go wrong with your pregnancy can be daunting and self-defeating. This section is provided as an educational reference. The chances that you will need it are slim, but if you do have problems in pregnancy, staying educated and informed can reduce related stress and help you take the best care of both baby and your body.

Gestational Diabetes

Gestational diabetes mellitus (diabetes of pregnancy) is caused by a problem with processing the glucose (blood sugar) in your bloodstream. Glucose is important to the body; it provides fuel for cellular growth and metabolism. To be processed effectively, glucose requires the companion hormone insulin. Insulin facilitates the transfer of glucose into the cells where the glucose is metabolized (processed for energy). If there is not enough insulin or if there is insulin that the body isn't using effectively, the result is a backup of glucose into the bloodstream, a situation that is potentially damaging to all of your organ systems and to a developing fetus.

When you develop gestational diabetes, your pancreas is still making plenty of insulin but your body isn't processing it efficiently. The condition, known as *insulin resistance*, is caused by certain placental hormones that counteract the effect of insulin (for example, estrogen, cortisol, and human placental lactogen, HPL). In most women, the condition doesn't reach critical levels and their blood sugar levels stay within normal ranges. In others, excess blood glucose accumulates to potentially dangerous levels and treatment is required.

Diagnosis and Treatment

Diagnosis of GDM is made with the oral glucose tolerance test (OGTT), given during weeks 24 to 28 of pregnancy.

Because blood sugar levels are influenced by dietary intake, your provider will probably try to treat your GDM with lifestyle and nutritional changes at the onset. A visit with a certified diabetes educator (CDE) and a registered dietitian (RD) can be invaluable in learning more about healthy menu planning, exercise, and the basics of blood sugar control.

You will have to self-test your blood glucose levels on a regular basis with a home meter. The home meter uses a lancet to prick your finger, arm, or another test site for a blood sample. The blood droplet is placed on a test reagent strip that goes into the meter, and the meter provides a blood glucose reading. Testing is generally recommended first thing in the morning (a fasting test) and after meals (postprandial)—usually at 1 hour and again at 2 hours after eating. Your doctor may recommend testing at additional times, such as after exercise, if he feels it is warranted. Refer to the table that follows to see the blood glucose levels that the American Diabetes Association recommends for women with gestational diabetes.

▼ BLOOD GLUCOSE LEVELS IN WOMEN WITH GESTATIONAL DIABETES

Test	Range
Fasting (before a meal)	<95 milligrams per deciliter, or mg/dL (5.3 millimoles per liter, or mmol/L)
1 hour postprandial (after meal)	<140 mg/dL (7.8 mmol/L)
2 hours postprandial (after meal)	<120 mg/dL (6.7 mmol/L)

If you don't experience significant improvement with dietary changes and your glucose levels still exceed normal ranges, you may have to use insulin injections to keep your blood sugar under control. Injections are typically done before meals to counteract their impact on glucose levels. Insulin does not cross the placenta and is not harmful to fetal development.

Possible Long-Term Health Effects

Without proper treatment, uncontrolled blood glucose levels can result in fetal death or in a condition known as *fetal macrosomia* (a baby that is abnormally large). Blood glucose crosses the placenta in high levels, and the fetus responds by producing more insulin to process the load. The extra glucose is ultimately stored as fat, and the baby potentially grows too large for vaginal birth.

Newborns of GDM moms may also suffer from hypoglycemia (low blood sugar) at birth as they are suddenly disconnected from the maternal surge of glucose and their high insulin production causes their blood glucose levels to plummet. They may also have an imbalance of blood calcium and blood magnesium levels at birth. Because of these risks, a neonatologist may be on the scene during labor and delivery to treat any potential complications.

Women who develop gestational diabetes have an increased risk of a diagnosis of type 2 diabetes later in life and should receive regular screening for the disease. Their children are also at risk for both type 2 diabetes and obesity. Fortunately, clinical studies have also shown that lifestyle changes involving regular exercise and a healthy diet can be extremely effective in preventing the onset of type 2 diabetes.

Hyperemesis Gravidarum

Hyperemesis gravidarum is excessive nausea and vomiting of pregnancy (that is, morning sickness) that goes beyond the normal gastrointestinal disturbance experienced by many women. Its exact cause is unknown. The condition is diagnosed when nausea and vomiting trigger one or more of the following symptoms:

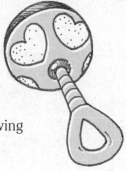

- ✓ Weight loss
- ✓ Ketosis/ketonuria
- ✓ Dehydration
- ✓ Electrolyte imbalance

Other conditions that can cause similar symptoms—including hyperthyroidism, pancreatitis, gall bladder or liver disease, gastritis, appendicitis, and ectopic pregnancy—should be ruled out before diagnosing hyperemesis gravidarum. Treatment typically involves intravenous therapy to rehydrate and encourage weight gain (parenteral nutrition). Hospitalization may be required, and medications may also be prescribed. Infants of mothers who experience this condition are more likely to have lower birth weights and to be small for gestational age.

Fortunately, hyperemesis gravidarum is relatively uncommon, occurring in less than 1 percent of pregnancies.

Incompetent Cervix

An incompetent cervix is a cervix that starts to painlessly open (thin and/or dilate) prematurely. The premature dilation is not associated with discomfort, contractions, or infection. It may be caused by genetic factors, family history, or prior surgeries.

As pregnancy progresses and your unborn child grows and places more pressure on the cervix, without treatment an incompetent cervix may result in miscarriage. Women who have had problems with incompetent cervix in previous pregnancies are generally offered a prophylactic (preventative) cerclage early in the second trimester. Cerclage is a minor surgical procedure to suture (stitch) the cervix closed, which may prevent premature cervical opening.

A cerclage may also be placed if you have signs of preterm cervical shortening on physical exam or by ultrasound. This is called a *rescue cerclage* and may be less effective than one placed prophylactically. Since it is a controversial topic and a high-risk situation, consultation with a high-risk OB doctor should be made. Women at risk for preterm labor—including those with multiples' gestations, those with previous preterm labor, and those with cervical and uterine abnormalities—are generally followed more closely throughout pregnancy.

Women with an incompetent cervix may be regularly monitored using transvaginal ultrasound to detect any cervical changes. Finally, bed rest may be prescribed to keep weight off your uterus, and abstinence from sexual intercourse will probably be recommended.

Intrauterine Growth Restriction (IUGR)

Intrauterine growth restriction (IUGR) occurs when fetal weight and size gains are estimated to be below the 10th percentile for gestational age. Some IUGR babies may be preterm, but others go to full term.

Possible causes of IUGR include:

✓ **Multiples' gestations.** IUGR occurs in at least one fetus in up to 20 percent of twins or higher-order multiples' pregnancies.

✓ **Infection.** Infectious agents such as toxoplasmosis and cytomegalovirus.

✓ **Placental problems.** Placenta previa, placenta accreta, or abruption, along with other placental abnormalities.

✓ **Maternal hypertension.** High blood pressure in pregnancy, including preeclampsia.

- ✓ **Maternal tobacco, alcohol, and drug use.** Smoking moms-to-be are almost twice as likely as nonsmokers to have low-birth-weight babies.

- ✓ **Poor maternal nutrition.** Malnutrition and inadequate protein intake can restrict fetal growth and may lead to adult health problems such as hypertension and insulin resistance.

- ✓ **Genetic anomalies.** Arrested physical and mental growth is one of the features of many chromosomal disorders, including Down syndrome and Edwards syndrome (trisomy 21 and trisomy 18).

- ✓ **Birth defects.** Birth defects such as a congenital heart or kidney malformation may restrict blood flow and affect fetal growth.

- ✓ **Altitude.** The reduced oxygen supply at high elevations decreases blood flow to the uterus and placenta and is thought to be a factor in IUGR and low birth weight.

- ✓ **Certain chronic illnesses.** Maternal heart disease, sickle cell disease, diabetes, and systemic lupus erythematosus (SLE, or lupus), among others.

A fundal height (uterus height) that is measuring too small for the due date is the first tip-off to IUGR. An ultrasound can give your provider an idea of actual fetal size, and if IUGR is diagnosed you will probably be undergoing regular ultrasounds, nonstress tests, and biophysical profiles through the remainder of pregnancy to follow your baby's progress.

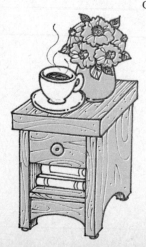

IUGR pregnancies are at risk for intrapartum asphyxia (blocked oxygen flow to fetus), oligohydramnios (low amniotic-fluid volume), and possible preterm birth and its related complications. At birth, IUGR babies are at risk for a number of medical problems, including high blood pressure, hypoglycemia (low blood sugar), anemia, polycythemia (an excess of red blood cells), neurological problems, and jaundice. Later in life they may experience some developmental problems. Low birth weight (LBW), including both IUGR and preterm LBW, is the leading cause of infant mortality in the United States.

IUGR that begins early in pregnancy and affects the fetal body uniformly is said to be *symmetric*. Symmetric IUGR may be caused by genetic abnormality, fetal infection, or exposure to a teratogen. Growth restriction that occurs later in pregnancy and is thought to be caused by insufficient fetal nutrition is termed *asymmetric IUGR*. It is also called *head-sparing IUGR* because the fetus has focused its limited resources on vital brain development, making the head in these babies much larger than the body. Asymmetric IUGR infants typically have a better prognosis or long-term outlook.

Placenta Problems

The placenta provides nourishment, blood, and oxygen to your baby and is literally what connects the two of you. Problems can occur with either the structure or the placement of the placenta and may pose a risk to you and to your unborn child.

Uteroplacental Insufficiency (UPI)

Uteroplacental insufficiency (UPI) occurs when the blood flow and consequently oxygen supply from mother to fetus are impaired or inadequate in some way. This is usually the result of an acute or chronic maternal illness (for example, hypertension, diabetes, preeclampsia, kidney disease), although it can arise from chromosomal abnormalities in the fetus. It may also occur in cases of multiples' gestation (twins, triplets, or more).

Clinical signs that UPI may be present include:

✓ **Oligohydramnios.** Low levels of amniotic fluid, apparent on ultrasound.

✓ **A nonreactive nonstress test (NST).** If the fetus is hypoxic (getting insufficient oxygen), its heart rate will not accelerate with (react to) fetal movement.

✓ **Late decelerations in a stress test (contraction stress test).** A slowdown in fetal heart rate that peaks toward the end of a contraction also indicates hypoxia.

✓ **Intrauterine growth restriction (IUGR; see above).** A fetus that is small for gestational age on ultrasound.

If you are diagnosed with UPI, steps will be taken to correct or treat the underlying cause, if possible. Fetal distress may be cause for immediate cesarean delivery.

Placenta Previa

A placenta that implants and grows near or covering the cervical opening (or cervical os) is called *placenta previa*. Placenta previa often resolves itself as the uterus enlarges (about 90 percent of the time). However, if it persists late in pregnancy, potentially life-threatening hemorrhage can occur when the cervix starts to efface (thin) and dilate (open).

Placenta previa may be total (completely covering the os), partial (partially covering the os), or marginal (on the margin, the edge, of the os). The condition is diagnosed by ultrasound. Vaginal bleeding is a possible symptom, but some women have no symptoms whatsoever.

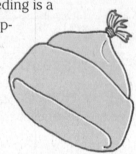

If bleeding does occur, bed rest may be prescribed. A blood transfusion may also be necessary. Women who have a placenta previa will usually require a cesarean delivery.

Low-Lying Placenta

A low-lying placenta is a placenta that is near the os but not close enough to be considered marginal. Like placenta previa, this type of placental implantation has a higher risk of bleeding during late pregnancy.

If you are diagnosed with a low-lying placenta in the first or second trimester, there's a good chance that the placenta will reposition itself as the uterus expands. Because the cervix begins to thin (efface) during the third trimester, if the placenta remains low in the uterus, hemorrhage becomes a risk. Women who still have a low-lying placenta in the third trimester are usually prescribed bed rest, and a cesarean section may be recommended.

Placental Abruption

Vaginal bleeding, abdominal cramping, and symptoms of shock (irregular heartbeat, low blood pressure, pale complexion) in the second and third trimesters may indicate that the placenta has begun to prematurely separate from the wall of the uterus—a condition called *placental abruption (abruptio placentae)*. Risk factors for placental abruption include maternal high blood pressure, cocaine use, or physical trauma to the abdomen.

Abruption may occur anytime after week 20, and if you have had a previous occurrence in an earlier pregnancy, your risk of experiencing it again is increased. Placental abruption may cause major life-threatening hemorrhage, fetal distress or possibly death, and preterm labor. However, a swift diagnosis and initiation of treatment, including blood transfusion, IV fluids, and oxygen, can do much to improve outcomes. Immediate delivery, possibly by C-section, is indicated in the majority of cases but depends on the stability of both mother and fetus and the length of gestation. In some cases in which only a small segment of the placenta prematurely separates from the uterine wall, careful maternal and fetal monitoring and bed rest may carry a pregnancy safely to term.

Placenta Accreta

Placenta accreta occurs when the placenta implants or attaches to the myometrium (uterine muscle) instead of to the endometrium (uterine lining). Placenta accreta can be further categorized into two subtypes based on the extent of myometrium invasion: placenta increta and placenta percreta. With placenta increta, the placenta implants through the uterine lining and penetrates the uterine muscle. And with placenta percreta, the placenta attachment passes through the uterine wall and may extend into nearby organs, such as the bladder.

In pregnancy complicated by placenta accreta, the placenta does not easily separate from the uterine wall during the third stage of delivery, and postpartum hemorrhage (PPH) occurs. A postpartum blood transfusion, arterial embolization, or an emergency hysterectomy (surgical removal of the uterus) may be required to stop the bleeding and stabilize the patient. If you are diagnosed with this condition prior to delivery, it's important to discuss the possibility of a hysterectomy. In many clinical situations, a hysterectomy may be unavoidable, but if an option is available, your doctor needs to know of any desire for more children so that she can preserve your fertility if at all possible.

Placenta accreta is more likely to occur in women with a history of cesarean delivery (and climbs with each subsequent C-section). In addition, women who are diagnosed with placenta previa have a substantially increased risk of placenta accreta.

If you are considered at risk for the condition, magnetic resonance imaging (MRI) and ultrasound may be used to confirm a diagnosis. A high alpha-fetoprotein (AFP) level may also be a sign of placenta accreta.

Preeclampsia/Eclampsia

Gestational hypertension (otherwise uncomplicated high blood pressure of pregnancy occurring after 20 weeks of gestation) appears in up to 10 percent of pregnancies. When high blood pressure in pregnancy is accompanied by proteinuria (protein in the urine) and edema (swelling), it is known as *preeclampsia*. Symptoms of preeclampsia include:

- ✓ High blood pressure (140/90 or higher)
- ✓ Excessive swelling of hands and/or feet
- ✓ Sudden weight gain
- ✓ Protein in the urine
- ✓ Blurry vision
- ✓ Abdominal pain (usually on the upper right side)
- ✓ Headache

Preeclampsia typically happens in the third trimester. If characterized as mild, it may be controlled by bed rest, medication, and careful monitoring of the fetus. Hospitalization may be required. If the pregnancy has reached week 37, delivery may be induced or performed via C-section to avoid further risk.

If the preeclampsia worsens or is severe, delivery may be required earlier than week 37. In some cases seizures may develop, indicating that preeclampsia has progressed to eclampsia. Eclampsia is rare but potentially life threatening, and your physician will weigh the risks and benefits to you and your baby when deciding when delivery is right in preterm pregnancies.

Premature Labor

Delivery of your baby after week 20 and before week 37 of pregnancy is considered preterm or premature. In cases of very early preterm labor when fetal lung maturity hasn't been established, your provider will probably try to delay the delivery for as long as possible. Preemies can suffer from a wide range of physical, neurological, and developmental difficulties, so any extra time spent in the womb is beneficial.

Are You At Risk?

A number of environmental and physical factors have been associated with an increased chance of preterm delivery. These include but are not limited to:

- Previous premature labor
- Pregnant with multiples (twins or more)
- Brief period of time between pregnancies
- Previous uterine surgery
- Hypertension (high blood pressure)
- Cigarette smoking
- Diagnosed incompetent cervix
- Drug or alcohol abuse
- Vaginal or systemic infection
- Obesity
- Being underweight prepregnancy
- Blood clotting disorders
- Exposure to the drug DES (diethylstilbestrol, a synthetic hormone)
- Domestic violence
- Lack of appropriate prenatal care
- Working more than 40 hours a week and/or standing more than 6 hours per day

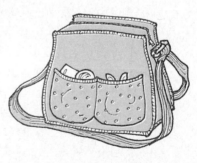

Women at high risk for preterm birth may be given the hormone progesterone, administered in the second and third trimesters, to cut the risk of preterm labor.

Warning Signs

If you experience any of the following warning signs of preterm labor, call your health care provider immediately. If you are out of town or unable to get in touch with her for any reason, go directly to the nearest hospital emergency room. With prompt action, it may be possible to delay your labor until your unborn child has adequate time to develop.

Symptoms include:

- ✓ Painful contractions at regular intervals
- ✓ Abdominal cramps
- ✓ Lower-back ache
- ✓ Bloody vaginal discharge
- ✓ Stomach pain
- ✓ Any type of fluid leak (large or small) from the vagina

Treatment

Preterm labor may be halted by bed rest, tocolytic medications (drugs that stop contractions), and intravenous hydration. Depending on your medical history and how far along your pregnancy is, you may be hospitalized. Home bed rest may also be prescribed, and you might be required to hook up to a fetal monitor on a regular basis. If preterm labor occurs between 24 and 34 weeks, corticosteroids may be administered as well, to hasten fetal lung surfactant development.

If your cervix dilates to 4 or 5 centimeters or if your fetus is showing signs of distress, preterm delivery may be unavoidable.

A "Level III" neonatal intensive care unit (NICU) is the best place for your newborn to receive treatment if he is delivered preterm. These units are highly experienced in the care of high-risk newborns and preemies and have state-of-the-art technology and training. The American Academy of Pediatrics and the American College of Obstetricians and Gynecologists recommend that all deliveries that occur earlier than week 32 take place at these facilities.

Preterm Premature Rupture of Membranes (PPROM)

Premature rupture of the amniotic membrane is not necessarily a problem if it occurs late in pregnancy. However, when it happens before week 37 of gestation, certain steps should be taken to ensure that your fetus has enough time for development in the womb.

PPROM may occur in women at risk for preterm labor. Other possible causes of PPROM include cervical incompetence and vaginal infection. If PPROM occurs prior to week 32, bed rest and frequent fetal heart monitoring may be recommended in an effort to prolong pregnancy until the fetal lungs mature. Antibiotics are administered to ward off infection in both fetus and mother, and steroids may be prescribed to speed lung surfactant production in the fetus. If PPROM occurs after weeks 34 or 35, your physician will probably recommend inducing your labor because the risks of infection are usually higher than the risks of a premature delivery.

Choroid Plexus Cysts

Ultrasound technology has become so advanced in recent years that it is able to pick up more anomalies earlier and earlier, anomalies that statistically tend to mean nothing in most low-risk pregnancies. One of these anomalies may be choroid plexus cysts—small cysts appearing on the choroid of the fetal brain. If no other abnormalities are seen on the scan, choroid plexus cysts have an excellent chance of resolving themselves by around week 24 with no ill effects to your child. The cysts are of note because in a small number of cases they have been associated with the serious chromosomal abnormality trisomy 18 (Edwards syndrome). A meeting with a genetic counselor will help you weigh the risks and benefits of further testing in your particular situation.

Ectopic Pregnancy

Ectopic pregnancy occurs when implantation takes place outside of the endometrial lining. In the majority of cases, it occurs in the Fallopian tube, which is why it is often referred to as a *tubal pregnancy*. However, an ectopic pregnancy may also implant in the ovary, cervix, abdominal cavity, or cornual portion of the uterus (close to the Fallopian tubes).

Unfortunately, pregnancy implantation must occur in the endometrium of the uterus for a pregnancy to safely continue. Allowing a pregnancy to progress in the Fallopian tube or other ectopic site will result in tubal or other rupture in the first trimester, unavoidable fetal death, and potential maternal death. If you are diagnosed with an ectopic pregnancy, it will need to be surgically removed or treated with the drug methotrexate (to induce medical abortion). Early treatment can preserve your fertility for subsequent pregnancies.

Women who have had previous ectopic pregnancies, who become pregnant with an IUD contraceptive device in place, who have a history of endometriosis and/or pelvic inflammatory disease (PID), and who have had a tubal ligation procedure are at a higher risk for ectopic pregnancy.

Early signs of ectopic pregnancy include low hCG levels or abnormally rising hCG levels (hCG should approximately double every 2 days in a normal pregnancy), abdominal pain, and irregular bleeding. An abdominal or transvaginal ultrasound can usually confirm the diagnosis. If it remains undiagnosed, ectopic pregnancy is potentially life threatening and can endanger future fertility. Warning signs that an undetected ectopic pregnancy may have ruptured include:

- ✓ Severe abdominal and/or pelvic pain
- ✓ Vaginal bleeding
- ✓ Dizziness
- ✓ Shoulder pain
- ✓ Nausea and vomiting

If you experience any of these symptoms, seek medical care immediately.

Molar Pregnancy

Like an ectopic pregnancy, a molar pregnancy is not viable. However, in a molar pregnancy, the implantation site is normal but the embryo is not. Called a *hydatidiform mole*, this placental tissue develops into a mass of cysts that are often described as resembling a cluster of grapes. There are two types of molar pregnancy: complete and incomplete (partial).

A complete molar pregnancy occurs when an egg with no genetic material inside is fertilized by one or two sperm. Most have forty-six chromosomes, all from the father (paternal). The pregnancy itself contains placental mass only and no embryonic tissue.

A partial molar pregnancy will usually contain some embryonic or fetal tissue. The majority of partial molar cases have two sets of paternal chromosomes and a single set of maternal chromosomes (sixty-nine in total).

Symptoms of molar pregnancy include:

✓ Too small or too large uterus for date
✓ Enlarged ovaries
✓ Possible high hCG levels
✓ Dark-brown bleeding in the first trimester
✓ Preeclampsia and toxemia

Ultrasound can make a diagnosis of molar pregnancy. Older women have a higher risk for the condition, and the risk of a subsequent molar pregnancy increases with each occurrence.

Removal by dilation and curettage (D&C) is the typical treatment for molar pregnancy. D&C is a surgical procedure involving dilating the cervix and suctioning the contents of the uterus. Synthetic hormones (oxytocin) may be administered during the procedure to induce uterine contractions.

A molar pregnancy has the potential to develop into a rare type of cancer known as *choriocarcinoma*. A chest x-ray, blood work, and other radiological exams are done prior to D&C to determine if the cancer has metastasized (spread to other parts of the body).

Follow-up blood tests may be required for 6 months to a year afterwards to ensure that hCG levels have returned to normal. Levels that fail to return to normal or start to rise are an indication that persistent gestational trophoblastic disease (GTD) is present and further treatment is necessary. Rarely, GTD may develop into choriocarcinoma. To accurately screen for these possibilities and ensure an early diagnosis, subsequent pregnancy should be avoided until the follow-up period is complete. Survival and remission rates are good if GTD is caught early and treated appropriately.

Miscarriage

A miscarriage that occurs before week 20 of gestation may be referred to as a spontaneous abortion or a missed abortion. Nearly 15 percent of all detected pregnancies miscarry. Approximately half of all miscarriages are caused by chromosomal or genetic abnormalities, while in the other half the cause remains unclear.

Other factors to be considered in a miscarriage are:

- Hormonal deficiencies
- Abnormalities of the cervix or uterus
- Incompatible blood types or Rh factor
- Viruses and infections
- Immune disorders

Warning Signs

Some of the warning signs of miscarriage can also happen in perfectly normal and healthy pregnancies. Light blood spotting, for example, is a common occurrence in pregnancy when implantation takes place. Do take any symptoms seriously and contact your provider as soon as they occur, but keep in mind that the appearance of blood spots or minor cramping doesn't guarantee miscarriage.

Signs and symptoms of miscarriage may include:

✓ Bright-red vaginal bleeding
✓ Abdominal cramping
✓ Low-back pain
✓ High fever

- ✓ Extreme nausea and vomiting that's sudden and unusual
- ✓ Amniotic fluid leakage
- ✓ Severe headache

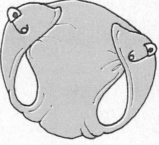

Some women panic when they experience a sudden improvement in previously troublesome pregnancy symptoms. Remember that this is a common phenomenon toward the end of the first trimester as hormone levels start to balance out. If you're still concerned or something just doesn't feel quite right, call your provider to schedule a quick appointment for a listen to the fetal heartbeat. Most will be happy to comply to ease your mind.

Coping with Loss

It doesn't take long to fall hopelessly in love with your unborn child, to dream about your future together, and to start making a special place within your family for him or her. "Love at first thought" is perhaps the most accurate way to describe the way many moms and dads feel about it.

That is what makes pregnancy loss so difficult at any point in the process. You may hear insensitive comments like "Well, at least you were only a few weeks along"—comments that are meant to be sympathetic but only serve to minimize the very real grief you are experiencing. Give yourself adequate time to mourn and to deal with the feelings of anger, guilt, frustration, and depression. Talk to your doctor about a referral to a pregnancy-loss support group or to a one-on-one counselor or therapist. You may also want to visit the Hygeia Foundation, Inc. and Institute for Perinatal Loss for online support and information, at *www.drberman.org/hygeiafoundation/*.

It's extremely important to take care of yourself during this difficult time. If you hadn't yet told anyone about the pregnancy at the point miscarriage occurred, it may be tougher to find enough time to reflect and grieve. Allow yourself to take a few sick or personal days off of work to spend healing time with your significant other and family. Don't rush things.

Trying Again

When to try again is a delicate issue. You need to be ready both emotionally and physically. Make sure you have had time to grieve your loss, and consult with your provider about the causes behind your first miscarriage. Your provider might recommend that you wait for a period to allow your body time to recover. If you do want to try again immediately, make sure you express your wishes so that you both can prepare properly for the next time around.

Most miscarriages occur due to factors completely beyond anyone's control—like a defective egg or sperm, or implantation outside the endometrium. Other triggers, such as teratogen exposure, may be avoided with special precautions in pregnancy. Definitely speak with your health care provider about your concerns and any special instructions given your medical history (for example, activity restrictions).

If you've experienced repeated miscarriage, considered clinically to be three consecutive pregnancy losses before week 20, further investigation is in order before attempting another pregnancy. The cause can sometimes be determined by a pathological examination of the miscarried fetus or embryo. A meeting with a genetic counselor and a full preconception diagnostic workup to examine your Fallopian tubes, uterus, and other possible sites of a problem may also be recommended.

Birth Plan Checklist

Consider starting your birth plan with a short note to both your provider and the nursing staff who will be caring for you during labor and delivery. Explain your general wishes for a healthy and safe delivery, for joint decision-making should medical interventions be required, and for open communication throughout the process. Read Chapter 15 to learn more about birth plans. Then use this checklist as a guide to assembling the basics.

1. Where will the birth take place?
   - ☐ Hospital
   - ☐ Birthing center
   - ☐ Home
   - ☐ Other: _____
   _____

2. Who will be there for labor support?
   - ☐ Husband or significant other
   - ☐ Doula
   - ☐ Friend
   - ☐ Family member

3. Will any room modifications or equipment be required to increase your comfort mentally and physically?
   - ☐ Objects from home (for example, pictures, blanket, pillow)
   - ☐ Lighting adjustments
   - ☐ Music

   - ☐ Video or photos of birth
   - ☐ Other: _____
   _____

4. Any special requests for labor prep procedures?
   - ☐ Forego enema
   - ☐ Self-administer the enema
   - ☐ Forego shaving
   - ☐ Shave self
   - ☐ Heparin lock instead of routine IV line
   - ☐ Other: _____
   _____

5. Eating and drinking during labor.
   - ☐ Want access to a light snack
   - ☐ Want access to water, sports drink, or other appropriate beverage
   - ☐ Want ice chips
   - ☐ Other: _____
   _____

6. Do you want pain medication?

☐ Analgesic (for example, Stadol, Demerol, Nubain)

☐ Epidural (If so, is timing an issue?)

☐ Other: _____

_____

7. What nonpharmaceutical pain relief equipment might you want access to?

☐ Hydrotherapy (that is, shower, whirlpool)

☐ Warm compresses

☐ Birthing ball

☐ Other: _____

_____

8. What interventions would you like to avoid unless deemed a medical necessity by your provider during labor? Specify your preferred alternatives.

☐ Episiotomy

☐ Forceps

☐ Internal fetal monitoring

☐ Pitocin (oxytocin)

☐ Other: _____

_____

9. What would you like your first face-to-face encounter with baby to be like?

☐ Hold off on all nonessential treatment, evaluation, and tests for a specified time

☐ If immediate tests and evaluation are necessary, you, your partner, or another support person will accompany baby

☐ Want to nurse immediately following birth.

☐ Would like family members to meet baby immediately following birth

☐ Other: _____

_____

10. If a cesarean birth is required, what is important to you and your partner?

☐ Type of anesthesia (for example, general versus spinal block)

☐ Having partner or another support person present

☐ Spending time with baby immediately following procedure

☐ Bonding with baby in the recovery room

☐ Type of postoperative pain relief and nursing considerations

☐ Other: _____

_____

11. Do you have a preference for who cuts the cord and when the cut is performed?

☐ Mom

☐ Dad

☐ Provider

☐ Delay until cord stops pulsing

☐ Cord blood will be banked, so cut per banking guidelines

☐ Cut at provider's discretion

☐ Other: _____

_____

12. What kind of postpartum care will you and baby have at the hospital?

☐ Baby will room-in with mom

☐ Baby will sleep in the nursery at nights

☐ Baby will breastfeed

☐ Baby will bottle-feed

☐ Baby will not be fed any supplemental formula and/or glucose water unless medically indicated

☐ Baby will not be given a pacifier

☐ Other: _____

_____

13. Considerations for after discharge.

☐ Support and short-term care for siblings

☐ Support if you've had a cesarean

☐ Maternity leave

☐ Other: _____

_____

Estimated Due Date Table

This chart lists due dates by month. Find the month and date on which your last menstrual period began, and then look below that line to see what your estimated due date is.

If your last period was . . .	1/1	1/2	1/3	1/4	1/5	1/6	1/7	1/8
Then your EDD is . . .	10/8	10/9	10/10	10/11	10/12	10/13	10/14	10/15

If your last period was . . .	1/9	1/10	1/11	1/12	1/13	1/14	1/15	1/16
Then your EDD is . . .	10/16	10/17	10/18	10/19	10/20	10/21	10/22	10/23

If your last period was . . .	1/17	1/18	1/19	1/20	1/21	1/22	1/23	1/24
Then your EDD is . . .	10/24	10/25	10/26	10/27	10/28	10/29	10/30	10/31

If your last period was . . .	1/25	1/26	1/27	1/28	1/29	1/30	1/31	
Then your EDD is . . .	11/1	11/2	11/3	11/4	11/5	11/6	11/7	

If your last period was . . .	2/1	2/2	2/3	2/4	2/5	2/6	2/7	2/8
Then your EDD is . . .	11/8	11/9	11/10	11/11	11/12	11/13	11/14	11/15

If your last period was . . .	2/9	2/10	2/11	2/12	2/13	2/14	2/15	2/16
Then your EDD is . . .	11/16	11/17	11/18	11/19	11/20	11/21	11/22	11/23

If your last period was . . .	2/17	2/18	2/19	2/20	2/21	2/22	2/23	2/24
Then your EDD is . . .	11/24	11/25	11/26	11/27	11/28	11/29	11/30	12/1

If your last period was . . .	2/25	2/26	2/27	2/28				
Then your EDD is . . .	12/2	12/3	12/4	12/5				

If your last period was . . .	3/1	3/2	3/3	3/4	3/5	3/6	3/7	3/8
Then your EDD is . . .	12/6	12/7	12/8	12/9	12/10	12/11	12/12	12/13

If your last period was . . .	3/9	3/10	3/11	3/12	3/13	3/14	3/15	3/16
Then your EDD is . . .	12/14	12/15	12/16	12/17	12/18	12/19	12/20	12/21

If your last period was . . .	3/17	3/18	3/19	3/20	3/21	3/22	3/23	3/24
Then your EDD is . . .	12/22	12/23	12/24	12/25	12/26	12/27	12/28	12/29

If your last period was . . .	3/25	3/26	3/27	3/28	3/29	3/30	3/31	
Then your EDD is . . .	12/30	12/31	1/1	1/2	1/3	1/4	1/5	

If your last period was . . .	4/1	4/2	4/3	4/4	4/5	4/6	4/7	4/8
Then your EDD is . . .	1/6	1/7	1/8	1/9	1/10	1/11	1/12	1/13

If your last period was . . .	4/9	4/10	4/11	4/12	4/13	4/14	4/15	4/16
Then your EDD is . . .	1/14	1/15	1/16	1/17	1/18	1/19	1/20	1/21

If your last period was . . .	4/17	4/18	4/19	4/20	4/21	4/22	4/23	4/24
Then your EDD is . . .	1/22	1/23	1/24	1/25	1/26	1/27	1/28	1/29

If your last period was . . .	4/25	4/26	4/27	4/28	4/29	4/30		
Then your EDD is . . .	1/30	1/31	2/1	2/2	2/3	2/4		

If your last period was . . .	5/1	5/2	5/3	5/4	5/5	5/6	5/7	5/8
Then your EDD is . . .	2/5	2/6	2/7	2/8	2/9	2/10	2/11	2/12

If your last period was . . .	5/9	5/10	5/11	5/12	5/13	5/14	5/15	5/16
Then your EDD is . . .	2/13	2/14	2/15	2/16	2/17	2/18	2/19	2/20

If your last period was . . .	5/17	5/18	5/19	5/20	5/21	5/22	5/23	5/24
Then your EDD is . . .	2/21	2/22	2/23	2/24	2/25	2/26	2/27	2/28

If your last period was . . .	5/25	5/26	5/27	5/28	5/29	5/30	5/31	
Then your EDD is . . .	3/1	3/2	3/3	3/4	3/5	3/6	3/7	

If your last period was . . .	6/1	6/2	6/3	6/4	6/5	6/6	6/7	6/8
Then your EDD is . . .	3/8	3/9	3/10	3/11	3/12	3/13	3/14	3/15

If your last period was . . .	6/9	6/10	6/11	6/12	6/13	6/14	6/15	6/16
Then your EDD is . . .	3/16	3/17	3/18	3/19	3/20	3/21	3/22	3/23

If your last period was . . .	6/17	6/18	6/19	6/20	6/21	6/22	6/23	6/24
Then your EDD is . . .	3/24	3/25	3/26	3/27	3/28	3/29	3/30	3/31

If your last period was . . .	6/25	6/26	6/27	6/28	6/29	6/30		
Then your EDD is . . .	4/1	4/2	4/3	4/4	4/5	4/6		

If your last period was . . .	7/1	7/2	7/3	7/4	7/5	7/6	7/7	7/8
Then your EDD is . . .	4/7	4/8	4/9	4/10	4/11	4/12	4/13	4/14

If your last period was . . .	7/9	7/10	7/11	7/12	7/13	7/14	7/15	7/16
Then your EDD is . . .	4/15	4/16	4/17	4/18	4/19	4/20	4/21	4/22

If your last period was . . .	7/17	7/18	7/19	7/20	7/21	7/22	7/23	7/24
Then your EDD is . . .	4/23	4/24	4/25	4/26	4/27	4/28	4/29	4/30

If your last period was . . .	7/25	7/26	7/27	7/28	7/29	7/30	7/31	
Then your EDD is . . .	5/1	5/2	5/3	5/4	5/5	5/6	5/7	

If your last period was . . .	8/1	8/2	8/3	8/4	8/5	8/6	8/7	8/8
Then your EDD is . . .	5/8	5/9	5/10	5/11	5/12	5/13	5/14	5/15

If your last period was . . .	8/9	8/10	8/11	8/12	8/13	8/14	8/15	8/16
Then your EDD is . . .	5/16	5/17	5/18	5/19	5/20	5/21	5/22	5/23

If your last period was . . .	8/17	8/18	8/19	8/20	8/21	8/22	8/23	8/24
Then your EDD is . . .	5/24	5/25	5/26	5/27	5/28	5/29	5/30	5/31

If your last period was . . .	8/25	8/26	8/27	8/28	8/29	8/30	8/31	
Then your EDD is . . .	6/1	6/2	6/3	6/4	6/5	6/6	6/7	

If your last period was . . .	9/1	9/2	9/3	9/4	9/5	9/6	9/7	9/8
Then your EDD is . . .	6/8	6/9	6/10	6/11	6/12	6/13	6/14	6/15

If your last period was . . .	9/9	9/10	9/11	9/12	9/13	9/14	9/15	9/16
Then your EDD is . . .	6/16	6/17	6/18	6/19	6/20	6/21	6/22	6/23

If your last period was . . .	9/17	9/18	9/19	9/20	9/21	9/22	9/23	9/24
Then your EDD is . . .	6/24	6/25	6/26	6/27	6/28	6/29	6/30	7/1

If your last period was . . .	9/25	9/26	9/27	9/28	9/29	9/30		
Then your EDD is . . .	7/2	7/3	7/4	7/5	7/6	7/7		

If your last period was . . .	10/1	10/2	10/3	10/4	10/5	10/6	10/7	10/8
Then your EDD is . . .	7/8	7/9	7/10	7/11	7/12	7/13	7/14	7/15

If your last period was . . .	10/9	10/10	10/11	10/12	10/13	10/14	10/15	10/16
Then your EDD is . . .	7/16	7/17	7/18	7/19	7/20	7/21	7/22	7/23

If your last period was . . .	10/17	10/18	10/19	10/20	10/21	10/22	10/23	10/24
Then your EDD is . . .	7/24	7/25	7/26	7/27	7/28	7/29	7/30	7/31

If your last period was . . .	10/25	10/26	10/27	10/28	10/29	10/30	10/31	
Then your EDD is . . .	8/1	8/2	8/3	8/4	8/5	8/6	8/7	

If your last period was . . .	11/1	11/2	11/3	11/4	11/5	11/6	11/7	11/8
Then your EDD is . . .	8/8	8/9	8/10	8/11	8/12	8/13	8/14	8/15

If your last period was . . .	11/9	11/10	11/11	11/12	11/13	11/14	11/15	11/16
Then your EDD is . . .	8/16	8/17	8/18	8/19	8/20	8/21	8/22	8/23

If your last period was . . .	11/17	11/18	11/19	11/20	11/21	11/22	11/23	11/24
Then your EDD is . . .	8/24	8/25	8/26	8/27	8/28	8/29	8/30	8/31

If your last period was . . .	11/25	11/26	11/27	11/28	11/29	11/30		
Then your EDD is . . .	9/1	9/2	9/3	9/4	9/5	9/6		

- -

If your last period was . . .	12/1	12/2	12/3	12/4	12/5	12/6	12/7	12/8
Then your EDD is . . .	9/7	9/8	9/9	9/10	9/11	9/12	9/13	9/14

If your last period was . . .	12/9	12/10	12/11	12/12	12/13	12/14	12/15	12/16
Then your EDD is . . .	9/15	9/16	9/17	9/18	9/19	9/20	9/21	9/22

If your last period was . . .	12/17	12/18	12/19	12/20	12/21	12/22	12/23	12/24
Then your EDD is . . .	9/23	9/24	9/25	9/26	9/27	9/28	9/29	9/30

If your last period was . . .	12/25	12/26	12/27	12/28	12/29	12/30	12/31	
Then your EDD is . . .	10/1	10/2	10/3	10/4	10/5	10/6	10/7	

- -

Top 100 Baby Names of the Past Century*

Rank	Boys	Girls	Rank	Boys	Girls	Rank	Boys	Girls
1	James	Mary	36	Larry	Amy	71	Terry	Victoria
2	John	Patricia	37	Jacob	Angela	72	Jeremy	Kathryn
3	Robert	Elizabeth	38	Jonathan	Virginia	73	Willie	Jacqueline
4	Michael	Jennifer	39	Scott	Brenda	74	Sean	Andrea
5	William	Linda	40	Justin	Catherine	75	Ralph	Gloria
6	David	Barbara	41	Raymond	Pamela	76	Jesse	Teresa
7	Richard	Susan	42	Brandon	Katherine	77	Billy	Rose
8	Joseph	Margaret	43	Gregory	Christine	78	Bruce	Janice
9	Charles	Dorothy	44	Patrick	Nicole	79	Roy	Sara
10	Thomas	Jessica	45	Samuel	Janet	80	Austin	Mildred
11	Christopher	Sarah	46	Benjamin	Debra	81	Eugene	Julia
12	Daniel	Betty	47	Dennis	Carolyn	82	Bryan	Theresa
13	Matthew	Nancy	48	Jack	Rachel	83	Louis	Judy
14	Donald	Karen	49	Jerry	Samantha	84	Harry	Beverly
15	Paul	Lisa	50	Walter	Frances	85	Christian	Hannah
16	Anthony	Helen	51	Alexander	Heather	86	Wayne	Denise
17	Mark	Sandra	52	Douglas	Diane	87	Russell	Grace
18	George	Donna	53	Peter	Maria	88	Alan	Marilyn
19	Steven	Ashley	54	Henry	Joyce	89	Philip	Amber
20	Kenneth	Kimberly	55	Tyler	Julie	90	Howard	Danielle
21	Edward	Carol	56	Harold	Martha	91	Randy	Brittany
22	Andrew	Michelle	57	Aaron	Joan	92	Jordan	Jane
23	Brian	Amanda	58	Jose	Evelyn	93	Juan	Diana
24	Kevin	Melissa	59	Adam	Kelly	94	Bobby	Lori
25	Joshua	Laura	60	Zachary	Christina	95	Vincent	Kathy
26	Ronald	Emily	61	Carl	Alice	96	Ethan	Tammy
27	Timothy	Deborah	62	Nathan	Marie	97	Johnny	Tiffany
28	Jason	Stephanie	63	Arthur	Judith	98	Phillip	Crystal
29	Jeffrey	Rebecca	64	Kyle	Doris	99	Fred	Lillian
30	Gary	Ruth	65	Gerald	Ann	100	Craig	Phyllis
31	Ryan	Sharon	66	Lawrence	Jean			
32	Eric	Cynthia	67	Albert	Lauren			
33	Nicholas	Kathleen	68	Roger	Cheryl			
34	Stephen	Anna	69	Keith	Emma			
35	Frank	Shirley	70	Joe	Megan			

*Compiled by the U.S. Social Security Administration using Social Security card applications for live births between January 1911 and February 2010.

Frequently Asked Questions

Will the bottle of champagne I shared with my husband on the night we conceived our baby be harmful?

Put this night of celebration behind you and stop feeling guilty. Binge drinking or regular abuse of alcohol when you are pregnant can cause birth defects, but an isolated episode of too much champagne probably has not harmed your unborn baby.

Heavy drinking, including binges or daily use, is associated with congenital defects. Babies born with fetal alcohol syndrome (FAS) show retarded growth, have central nervous system problems, and characteristic facial features, including a small head, a thin upper lip, a short upturned nose, a flattened nasal bridge and a general underdeveloped look of the face. Because of the critical nervous system involvement, many show tremulousness, can't suck, are hyperactive, have abnormal muscle tone, and are later diagnosed with attention deficit disorder as well as mental retardation.

Relying on alcohol out of habit or cravings can also end your pregnancy abruptly. Heavy to moderate drinkers seem to experience a higher incidence of miscarriage in the second trimester, as well as problems with the placenta. Other complications linked to alcohol use are congenital heart defects, brain abnormalities, spinal and limb defects, and urinary and genital problems.

What should I take for a headache?

Most doctors say that aspirin is fine for most of your pregnancy. You should avoid it in the last month. Tylenol, or an analgesic based on acetaminophen, is also recommended for headaches, but be sure to ask your doctor before taking any medication during pregnancy.

I have terrible allergies. Is there anything my doctor is going to be able to recommend?

For some women, pregnancy can feel like a bad head cold. The increased volume of blood to your mucus membranes can make the lining of your respiratory tract swell. You may even experience nosebleeds. Fortunately, there are safe medications available to ease the symptoms, so consult with your doctor. See about taking extra vitamin C. A humidifier can also be helpful. If you experience nosebleeds as a result of allergies, try packing the nostril with gauze and then pinching your nose between your thumb and forefinger. To shrink the blood vessels and reduce bleeding, try putting an ice pack on your nose.

If I develop an infection, are there any antibiotics safe for expectant moms?

Yes. Pharmaceutical companies are coming up with new antibiotics all the time, and a number of them are safe for pregnancy. Many doctors believe that natural and synthetic penicillins are the safest antibiotics to take during pregnancy, so if you are not allergic to these oldest weapons against infection, you are definitely in luck. If you do get sick, make sure that your obstetrician is aware of anything your family doctor or another specialist may be prescribing.

What are the dangers of X-rays to my unborn baby?

According to the American Academy of Family Physicians (AAFP), the maximum safe fetal radiation dose during pregnancy is 5 rad, or the equivalent of 50,000 dental X-rays or 250 mammograms. CT scans, fluoroscopic studies, and nuclear medicine tests involve slightly higher doses than conventional X-rays, but in general still fall well within the range of acceptable exposure. In each case, the benefits of imaging need to be weighed against the potential risk to the fetus, and if at all possible, tests involving radiation should be avoided in the first trimester of pregnancy.

Can ultrasounds give misleading information?

While it's possible that you may be having a baby boy even if his external sex organs aren't visible in the ultrasound and therefore you may incorrectly think you are having a girl, most technicians won't state your baby's gender unless they are absolutely certain. If the sonogram indicates a due date that seems wrong, you might ask, "Could I possibly have dated the start of my pregnancy incorrectly?" Experts say that an ultrasound done at sixteen weeks is more accurate in regards to gestational age than an ultrasound done later in your pregnancy. When dating the length of a pregnancy, the ultrasound technician can be accurate within a few days. Ultrasounds date your pregnancy from the point of conception, which is a few days different from the point of your last period. Later ultrasounds are more accurate when determining your baby's gender. A very clear image must be obtained for the ultrasound to determine whether you are expecting a boy or a girl, and this may be more difficult to see in the early stages.

Why do I feel so hot and sweaty?

Your metabolism works overtime during pregnancy. Your body is burning more calories, and as a result, you often feel warm. An increase in blood supply to the surface of your skin, as well as hormones, all have an effect on how hot you feel. Keep cool by dressing in natural fibers and layering clothes so that you can always cool off by removing a layer. Hop in the shower; pat on a little talcum powder afterwards. You may need to change antiperspirants if your normal brand isn't working. To avoid dehydration as your body is working hard to burn calories and produce more blood, drink plenty of water.

Why do I often feel scatterbrained?

Increased hormones can make your thinking a bit foggy—just as they can during your menstrual cycle. Manage the situation by reducing your stress load, making lists, and going easy on yourself.

What is toxoplasmosis, and should I worry about getting it?

Toxoplasmosis is rare, but it is a virus that can affect your baby in the womb. When cats are allowed to run freely outside they can end up with a parasite that settles in the intestines and is passed on through cat feces. Toxoplasmosis can cause brain damage and other medical problems in your unborn child. Cats also frequent gardens and sandboxes, so wear gloves and wash your hands thoroughly after being outside. Don't clean any litter boxes during your pregnancy (ask your partner or a friend to help you).

My doctor recommends lots of iron, but it makes me feel nauseated. What should I do?

Take iron-rich prenatal vitamin supplements between meals with plenty of water or along with a fruit juice rich in vitamin C, which enhances the absorption of iron. Avoid drinking milk, coffee, or tea with your iron supple-

ments because these beverages inhibit iron absorption. Add liver, red meat, fish, poultry, enriched breads and cereals, green leafy vegetables, eggs, and dried fruits to your diet to increase dietary iron.

What kinds of food cravings are normal?

Many pregnant women crave sweet or salty foods. Cravings for nonfood items such as dirt, soap, ash, or coffee grounds are different. A phenomenon called pica, which has shown up in medical literature since the sixth century, results in strange cravings that can cause serious problems for a pregnant mother and her unborn baby. If you have a craving to eat clay, ashes, laundry starch, or other unusual substances, seek medical attention right away.

Does intercourse hurt the baby?

Unless you have a high-risk pregnancy, you are not going to harm your baby by having sex. Sex is quite safe in a normal pregnancy. Vaginal bleeding, a history of miscarriage or premature labor, or a diagnosis of placental problems are good reasons to restrict intercourse, however. During the last month before your due date, you also should proceed with caution. Ask your practitioner if you have any concerns.

Should I circumcise my baby?

The American Academy of Pediatrics takes the stance that there is currently no firm medical or hygienic ground for performing routine circumcision (removal of the foreskin that covers the head of the penis) in new-born boys. However, the AAP also cited the importance of weighing cultural and religious beliefs and considering the child's best interest when deciding whether or not to circumcise a newborn male. If circumcision is performed, analgesia can be used to relieve the pain.

How soon can I have sex after the baby's birth?

Many doctors recommend waiting four to six weeks before having intercourse. Very few couples are able to swing back into a sex life immediately after the birth of a baby. Keep in mind either way that you can get pregnant in the period following birth. You should get back into your contraceptive routine before the mood strikes. Your doctor can give you a prescription before you leave the hospital, if necessary.

I'm getting varicose veins in my legs. Is this common in pregnancy?

The hair-fine marks, also known as spider veins, usually appear on the lower legs and are caused when increased blood volume and pressure damage the valves that regulate blood flow up out of the blood vessels of the legs. The result is pooled blood in the vein and that telltale squiggly red or blue line.

Supportive stockings, putting your feet up, resting on your left side, and taking an occasional walk when you need to stand for long periods of time may relieve leg soreness associated with varicose veins.

I've had a miscarriage in the past. Is there a way to prevent it this time around?

Many miscarriages occur due to factors completely beyond anyone's control—a defective egg or sperm, or implantation outside of the endometrium. Other triggers, such as teratogen exposure, may be avoided with special precautions in pregnancy. Speak with your health care provider about your concerns and any special instructions given your medical history (such as restrictions on your activity).

What if I don't get to the hospital in time?

Every woman has heard stories of impatient babies being born in the backseats of taxicabs, but these impromptu deliveries are not common. Most women have plenty of time to make it to the hospital safe and sound; the average labor period runs twelve to fourteen hours. If you're concerned, you can take some basic precautions. Work out a route to the hospital in advance with your partner, keep your gas tank full, and have cash on hand for a cab just in case your car chooses the moment you go into labor to conk out.

If I'm overdue, will my provider induce me if I request it?

Whether or not to induce depends on a number of factors. Is the cervix effaced or dilated? Are you fairly sure your due date was accurate to begin with? Have you had a previous C-section? Have you had other complicating factors during pregnancy (e.g., placenta previa, umbilical cord prolapse)? Generally, if you've hit the thirty-nine-week mark, you have no history of C-section or other medical contraindications, and your provider thinks induction is indicated, she will schedule one for you.

What is umbilical cord blood banking?

Blood from the umbilical cord contains stem cells, those blank-slate cells from which all organs and tissues are built. Cord blood collected immediately after birth is placed in a collection kit and flown to a facility where it is cryogenically frozen and "banked" for later use if needed. The theory behind cord blood banking is that if your child ever develops a disease or condition requiring stem-cell treatment, the blood can be thawed and used for her treatment. If it matches certain biological markers, cord blood can be used to treat other family members as well. However, banking is cost prohibitive for many and requires an annual storage fee for as long as you would like the cord blood frozen. In recent years, some facilities have also made placenta blood banking available. The AAP has stated that "private storage of cord blood as "biological insurance" should be discouraged." Many experts recommend donating cord blood to a public cord blood bank instead.

I have splotches of discolored skin on my face and abdomen. Is this normal?

Yes. Pregnancy hormones can cause hyperpigmentation of your skin, which makes certain areas of your skin (most commonly around the forehead, nose, cheeks, abdomen, and areolas) to darken. These discolored spots are usually dark on light-skinned women and light on dark-skinned women. Don't worry, though—these discolored patches will fade and eventually go away after your baby is born.

Are there exercises I should avoid during pregnancy?

Yes. A few sports are considered inappropriate during any phase of pregnancy. Mostly these sports are dangerous for reasons related to balance and risk of physical blows. It is not recommended that pregnant women ride horses, scuba dive, downhill ski, play rugby, or engage in other contact sports.

How do I know if I'm doing Kegel exercises right?

If you are doing Kegels correctly, you will not be tightening other muscles like your buttocks or thighs. You will be isolating this internal muscle and not straining other ones in the process.

Will eating too much sugar during pregnancy lead to gestational diabetes?

No, eating too much sugar does not directly cause any type of diabetes. Diabetes is a disorder in which the body cannot properly utilize insulin or does not produce insulin, which regulates blood sugar levels. Gestational diabetes is the result of changing hormones within a woman's body.

Do folic acid supplements really make that much of a difference in preventing certain birth defects?

According to the United States Centers for Disease Control (CDC), when taken one month before conception and throughout the first trimester, folic acid supplements have been proven to reduce the risk of neural tube defects by 50–70 percent.

Can eating more than three times a day be part of a healthy diet?

Yes. For women who are pregnant or for anybody who enjoys a healthy lifestyle, eating several small meals during the day can fit nicely into a healthy eating pattern. It can help you to fit in those extra calories and food group servings without having to eat large meals all at once, which can be difficult for women who may be having a problem with nausea or morning sickness.

Is it okay to take a calcium supplement if I don't eat dairy foods?

If you can't get enough calcium from the foods you choose, a supplement can be a good idea. The rule of thumb should always be food before supplements, though. First, include calcium-containing foods in your diet as much as possible, and then supplement on top of that. Never let a supplement take the place of an entire food group or nutrient such as calcium.

Is it unhealthy to have an aversion to vegetables during my first trimester?

It is common for women to have food aversions even to healthy foods such as vegetables. Try drinking vegetable juice instead of eating whole vegetables. You can also eat more fruit, since many of them contain some of the same nutrients as vegetables. Keep taking your prenatal vitamins to ensure you are getting all of the nutrients that your body needs at this time. However, it's always best to get your nutrients from food before supplements. If you have a temporary aversion to a healthy food, make substitutions. If you're not sure what to substitute, be sure to speak to a dietitian.

How can I tell whether I am experiencing morning sickness or something more serious?

If you vomit more than three or four times a day, are hardly able to keep any food down, lose weight, feel very tired and dizzy, and urinate less than usual, you may have something more serious than run-of-the-mill morning sickness—specifically, you may be suffering from hyperemesis gravidarum (HG). Additional symptoms include increased heart rate, headaches, and pale, dry-looking skin. It is important to diagnose and treat HG as soon as possible, so contact your doctor if you feel any of these symptoms or feel that your morning sickness is more serious.

Index

A

Adjustments, making, 42–43, 283–89, 294–98

Alcohol risks, 102–4

Alpha-fetoprotein (AFP), 71, 73, 85

Amniocentesis, 48, 68, 71–74, 174

Amniotic fluid, 16, 70–74, 106, 158, 186, 209, 222

Amniotic sac, 16, 76, 161, 168, 170–76, 246

Analgesics, 235

Anesthesia, 202, 235–37, 243–45

Antepartum depression, 12. *See also* Depression

Apgar test, 248

Apgar, Virginia, 248

B

Baby
    birth plan for, 195–205
    bonding with, 283
    bottle-feeding, 257–58, 263–64
    breastfeeding, 250, 255–72
    breech position of, 211–12
    bringing home, 273–88
    burping, 264–65
    changes in, 293–94
    cost of having, 37–42, 91
    delivery of, 240–42

due dates for, 21–22, 228–29, 320–24

first contact with, 203–4, 241–42, 247–48

first trimester, 15–17, 47–49, 81–82

gender of, 48, 69, 72

heartbeat of, 75–76, 86

names for, 90, 325

pictures of, 199

screenings of, 248

second trimester, 105–7, 134, 159

sleep requirements for, 280

space for, 32–33, 215–16

third trimester, 184, 208, 220

"Baby blues," 280–82. *See also* Postpartum depression

Babyproofing home, 36–37

Bed rest, 214–15

Biophysical profile (BPP), 77

Birth control, 164, 275

Birthing center
    birth plan for, 195–205
    length of stay in, 249–50
    monitors in, 201, 233
    packing bags for, 225–26
    preregistration for, 201
    rooming in, 204–5, 249
    touring, 192

Birth plan, 195–205
    for birthing center, 195–205
    checklist for, 317–19
    creating, 195–97
    for cutting cord, 203
    family and, 199–200
    finalizing, 225
    interventions and, 202–3
    labor and, 200
    for pain relief, 201–2
    postpartum planning, 205

Birth Without Violence, 191

Blood pressure, 9, 60–63, 79, 94, 143, 160, 211, 244

Blood work, 63–66, 85–86

Body
    aches and pains, 134–38, 160, 185–87, 210–11
    exercising, 10, 112–15, 135–36, 290–91
    during first trimester, 17–20, 49–50, 56–57, 82–87
    during second trimester, 107–8, 134–35, 157, 159–60
    during third trimester, 184–87, 208–11, 220–22

Bonding, with baby, 283

Bonding, with partner, 43

Bottle-feeding
    basics of, 263–64
    costs of, 40

We Have

EVERYTHING®

on Anything!

With more than 19 million copies sold, the Everything® series has become one of America's favorite resources for solving problems, learning new skills, and organizing lives. Our brand is not only recognizable—it's also welcomed.

The series is a hand-in-hand partner for people who are ready to tackle new subjects—like you!

For more information on the Everything® series, please visit *www.adamsmedia.com*

The Everything® list spans a wide range of subjects, with more than 500 titles covering 25 different categories:

Business	History	Reference
Careers	Home Improvement	Religion
Children's Storybooks	Everything Kids	Self-Help
Computers	Languages	Sports & Fitness
Cooking	Music	Travel
Crafts and Hobbies	New Age	Wedding
Education/Schools	Parenting	Writing
Games and Puzzles	Personal Finance	
Health	Pets	